OXFORD MEDICAL

MW01480597

SLIDE INTERPRETATION

**in oral diseases
and the oral manifestations
of systemic diseases**

SLIDE INTERPRETATION

in oral diseases
and the oral manifestations
of systemic diseases

CRISPIAN SCULLY

Professor of Oral Medicine and Oral Surgery, University Department of Oral Medicine and Oral Surgery, Bristol.

and

JONATHAN SHEPHERD

Consultant Senior Lecturer in Oral and Maxillo-facial Surgery, University Department of Oral Medicine and Oral Surgery, Bristol

Oxford New York Tokyo

OXFORD UNIVERSITY PRESS

1986

Oxford University Press, Walton Street, Oxford OX2 6DP
Oxford New York Toronto
Delhi Bombay Calcutta Madras Karachi
Petaling Jaya Singapore Hong Kong Tokyo
Nairobi Dar es Salaam Cape Town
Melbourne Auckland
and associated companies in
Beirut Berlin Ibadan Nicosia

Oxford is a trade mark of Oxford University Press

Published in the United States
by Oxford University Press, New York

British Library Cataloguing in Publication Data
Scully, C. M.
Slide interpretation in oral diseases and the
oral manifestations of systemic diseases.
1. Mouth — Diseases   2. Teeth — Diseases
3. Oral manifestations of general diseases
4. Symptomatology
I. Title   II. Shepherd, Jonathan
617'.522'00222   RC815
ISBN 0-19-261497-5

Library of Congress Cataloging in Publication Data
Scully, Crispian.
Slide interpretation in oral diseases and the
oral manifestations of systemic diseases.
(Oxford medical publications)
Bibliography: p.
Includes index.
1. Teeth — Diseases.   2. Mouth — Diseases.
3. Oral manifestations of general diseases.   I. Shepherd,
Jonathan.   II. Title.   III. Series. [DNLM: 1. Mouth
Diseases — examination questions.   2. Oral Manifestations
— examination questions.   WU 18 S437s]
RK307.S38   1986   617'.5220758   85-15497
ISBN 0-19-261497-5

Set by Graphicraft Typesetters Ltd, Hong Kong
Printed in Hong Kong

Preface

It has become apparent from our teaching and examining of BDS, FDS, MBBS, and MGDS candidates in Bristol, Glasgow, Leeds, and London that one of the better ways of teaching and of examining a candidate's ability to manage clinical problems is by the presentation of data in slide form together with relevant questions. This type of examination is being increasingly used both in undergraduate and postgraduate dental examinations and has been popular in medicine for some years.

It has also become apparent that few medical students or graduates have any substantial degree of training at 'looking in the mouth' and yet it is to the medical practitioner that many patients turn, when they have oral disease.

Therefore we have produced this selection of clinical slides on oral diseases and oral manifestations of systemic disease in an attempt to be helpful to candidates for the BDS and MBBS examinations and also for MGDS and for the FDS and MRCP examinations.

Each section is a mixture of problems ranging from the common to the exotic and from simple dental lesions to oral lesions in systemic disease. The depth of knowledge required ranges from undergraduate to postgraduate level. The information given is not intended to be comprehensive and should be used to complement standard textbooks.

We hope, however, that this book will serve to stimulate and, perhaps, re-stimulate the neurons, if trying to absorb the standard texts becomes rather tiresome.

Bristol   C. S.
May 1985   J. P. S.

Acknowledgements

The slides used are from our collection and for this our greatest debt is to the patients and referring practitioners. Inevitably, we may have used some slides of patients who have been seen by others and certainly we are grateful to our previous chiefs, Professor D. K. Mason (Glasgow), Professor F. Hopper and Mr. D. P. Dyson (Leeds), Professor E. O. Adekeye (Kaduna) and Dr R. T. D. Emond (London). A few of the slides have already appeared in print, and we are particularly grateful to Update Publications for permission to re-use our slides here and to Professor R. A. Cawson (Guy's) who originally loaned slides 2.7 and 3.8. We are also grateful to Professor A.I. Darling and J. Fletcher for use of some slides from the Bristol collection. Nye Fathers has kindly helped with the preparation of the slides. Hugh Levers and Dimitris Malamos helped check the text. We are grateful to the staff of Oxford University Press who have encouraged us and been responsible for pursuing the book to completion.

Contents

PAPER 1

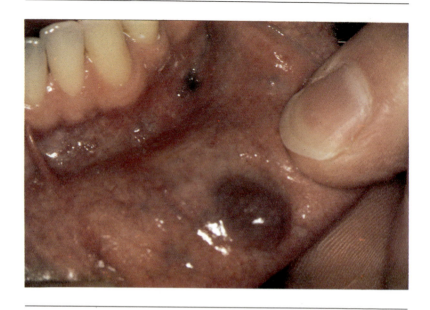

Q 1.1 (a) Two lesions are shown here. What are they?

(b) What is the aetiology of each lesion?

(c) What treatment may be indicated for each?

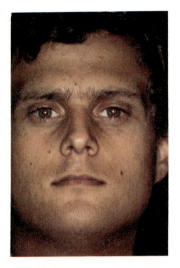
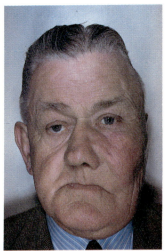

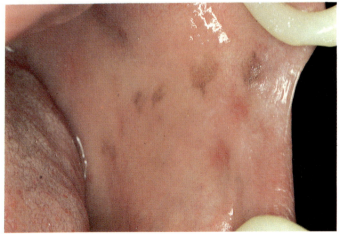

Q 1.2   (a) The patient on the left complained of hyperpigmentation (the
             older patient is shown for comparison). The oral photograph is
             from the pigmented patient. What disorder must be excluded?

        (b) What are the typical symptoms of this disease?

        (c) What are the clinical and laboratory findings?

        (d) What special precautions should be taken when such a patient
             attends for surgical removal of an impacted lower third molar
             under local anaesthesia?

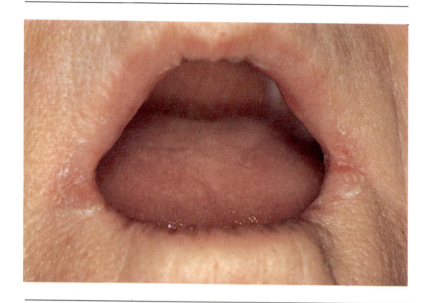

Q 1.3 (a) What is this condition?

(b) What are possible causes?

(c) What micro-organisms may be isolated?

(d) If this is seen in a child what would you do?

(e) How would you manage the patient illustrated?

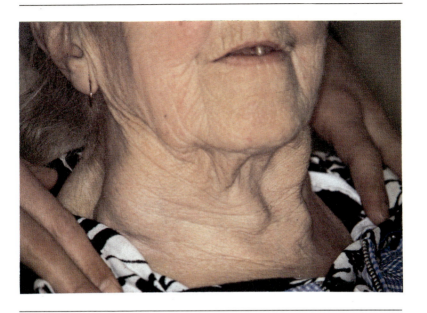

Q 1.4   (a) What is the possible cause of these swellings?

(b) How would you investigate this patient?

(c) Give a differential diagnosis.

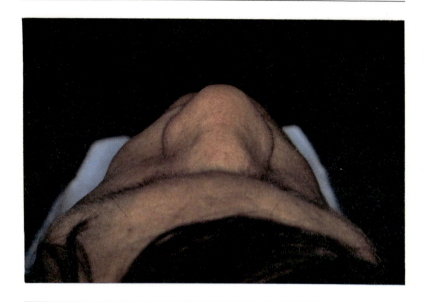

Q 1.5 This 23 year old man complained of a facial asymmetry, but questioning did not reveal a history of trauma over the past year.

(a) What abnormality affecting the right side of the face is illustrated here?

(b) What are the likely causes?

(c) How may this be managed?

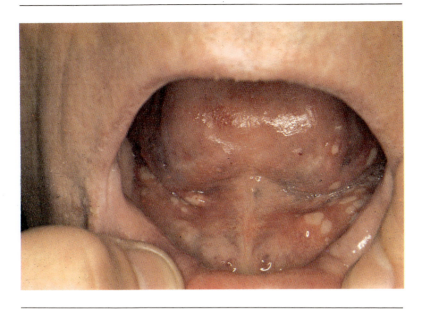

Q 1.6   (a) What type of recurrent oral ulceration is this?

(b) What are the other types?

(c) What local treatments are available?

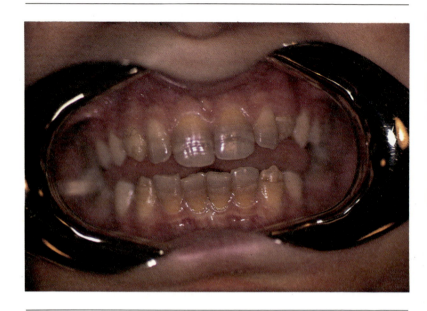

Q 1.7 (a) What is shown here?

(b) What else should be considered about the patient's medical condition?

(c) What treatment is indicated?

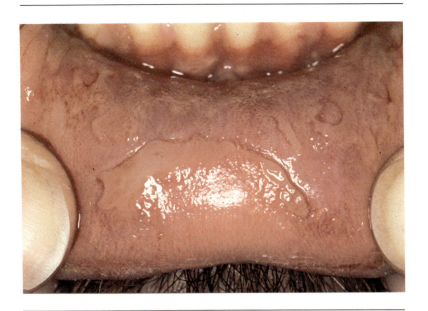

Q 1.8   These are the oral lesions in a 29 year old male who had had a persistently sore mouth for 2 years. The only other findings of note were an iron deficiency anaemia and positive occult blood in the stool.

(a) What is the likely cause of his anaemia?

(b) How would you investigate his gastro-intestinal tract?

(c) Which three important gastro-intestinal disorders may be associated with oral ulcers?

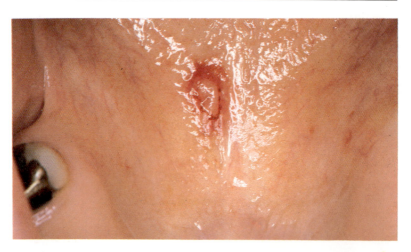

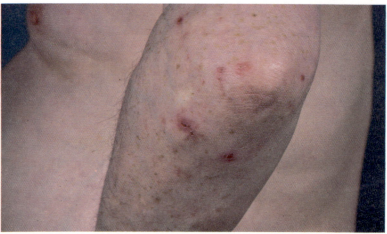

Q 1.9 These are the oral lesions in a 49 year old male who admitted to a pruritic rash as shown here.

   (a) What is the most common disorder in which oral and pruritic cutaneous lesions may be associated?

   (b) What is the probable diagnosis in this patient?

   (c) What, if any, are the characteristic immunofluorescent findings?

   (d) What is the management?

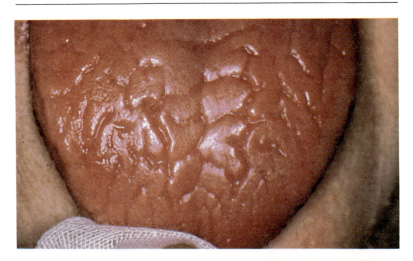

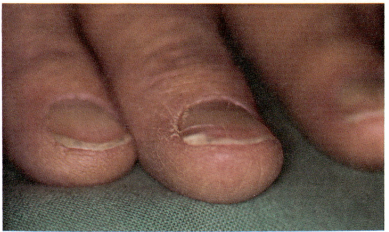

Q 1.10 This elderly patient complained of a persistently burning sensation in the tongue.

   (a) What is the term for this appearance of the tongue?

   (b) If there was also oral ulceration and angular cheilitis, what would you suspect?

   (c) The same patient had this appearance of his nails. What is the probable diagnosis?

   (d) What are likely to be the most useful investigations?

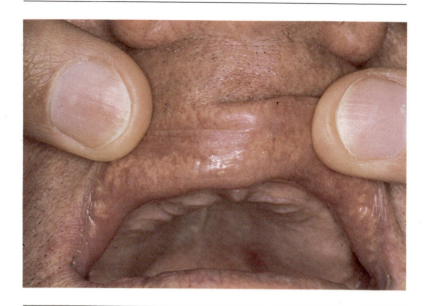

Q 1.11 This patient was referred with a diagnosis of thrush that had failed to respond to nystatin.

   (a) What comments would you make about that diagnosis?

   (b) What would be seen histologically?

   (c) How should this patient be treated?

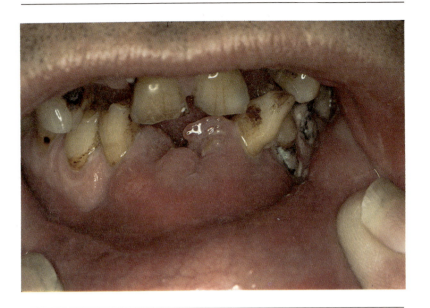

Q 1.12 This 55 year old publican presented with a firm swelling in the anterior mandible together with loosening and loss of lower incisor teeth. His medical history revealed a chronic cough, productive of blood.

(a) What should be considered in the differential diagnosis?

(b) How would you investigate this patient?

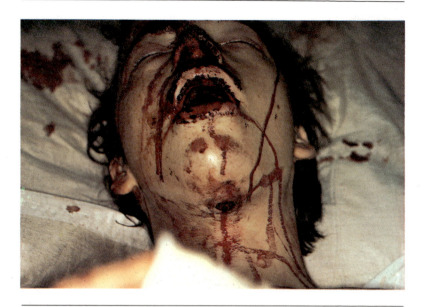

Q 1.13 This 20 year old man was brought to hospital having sustained a low velocity type (handgun) gunshot wound. The entry wound is situated in the submental region and the exit wound in the midline frontal region below the hairline.

(a) Outline the principles of primary management in this type of case.

(b) How do high velocity missile wounds differ from the type of injury illustrated here?

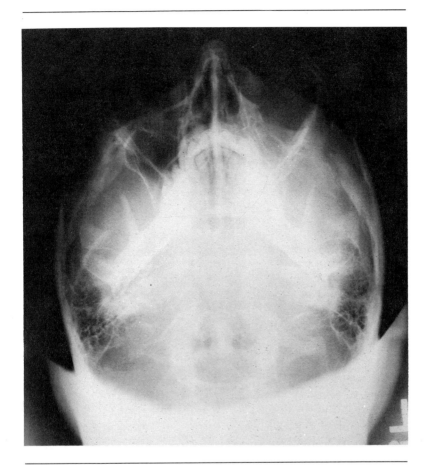

Q 1.14 (a) Which radiographic view is this?

(b) Which abnormalities are illustrated in this radiograph?

(c) What is the diagnosis?

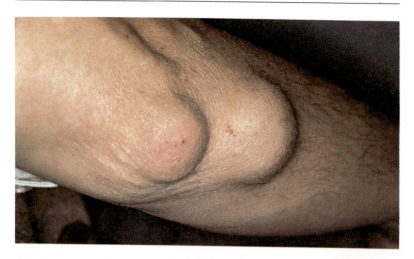

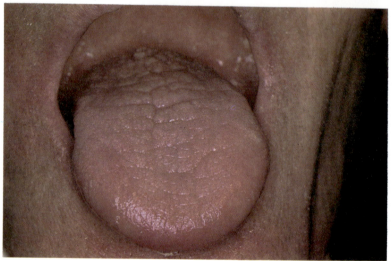

Q 1.15 This 59 year old man complained of a sore tongue, itching eyes, and joint pains.

(a) What is the probable predisposing cause of the sore tongue?

(b) Which blood tests are the most useful in confirming the diagnosis?

(c) What are the oral complications of the condition shown?

A 1.1   (a) (i)   Amalgam tattoo in buccal sulcus. These lesions are nearly always macular and dark blue or black in colour and affect mucosa adjacent to an amalgam-restored tooth.

        (ii)   Cavernous haemangioma in lip.

    (b) (i)   Traumatic implantation of amalgam particles into the tissues during restoration of a tooth. Amalgam tatoos *MAY* show radiopacity on a radiograph.

        (ii)   Haemangiomas are hamartomatous lesions which manifest themselves at birth or within the first few years of life. Raised lesions such as this example are frequently traumatized and sometimes give rise to prolonged bleeding. Some authorities believe that these lesions are benign neoplasms. Clinical diagnosis is based on the fact that they empty on pressure.

    (c) (i)   Normally no treatment is required for an amalgam tattoo but simple surgical excision is sometimes indicated for comestic reasons, or to exclude a melanoma or other pigmented lesion (see A1.2).

        (ii)   Elimination of cavernous haemangiomas may be achieved by a variety of means. Surgical excision has the disadvantage that troublesome bleeding may be a feature and that considerable scarring may accompany the excision of a large lesion. An advantage of surgical excision is that the resulting specimen can be examined histologically if there is any doubt about the diagnosis. Cryosurgical and electrosurgical methods do not normally allow this.

Endothelium is highly susceptible to low temperature injury which will also cause stasis in the abnormal vascular channels. Cryosurgery is therefore an excellent treatment for these lesions and, due to the preservation of the normal connective tissue fibre network, little scarring is produced. Cryosurgery may be performed without recourse to local or general anaesthesia but is, however, followed by a lengthy healing period as compared with surgical excision. Electrosurgery has its advocates in the management of small haemangiomas, but this technique is sometimes followed by pronounced post-operative scarring as well as troublesome bleeding during the procedure. Laser therapy using the argon laser may be valuable — especially in accessible superficial haemangiomas.

A 1.2   (a) Addison's disease or primary hypoadrenocorticism. This is characterized by atrophy of the adrenal cortices and failure of secretion of cortisol and aldosterone. Usually there are circulating autoantibodies to the adrenal cortex in autoimmune hypoadrenocorticism. Other rare causes include adrenal tuberculosis, histoplasmosis, malignancy, haemorrhage, sarcoidosis, and amyloidosis. In addition to the hyperpigmentation seen here, weight loss, weakness, hypotension, anorexia, and nausea may also be features.

The hyperpigmentation is due to melanin. Low serum cortisol levels stimulate the pituitary gland to produce increased amounts of adrenocorticotrophic hormone (ACTH) which acts as a melanocyte stimulating hormone.

Oral pigmentation in Addison's disease is usually an early sign and is brown or black, predominantly at the occlusal line in the buccal mucosa, but also elsewhere.

Oral pigmentation is usually racial in origin. The implantation of dental amalgam may produce amalgam tattoos (see A1.1) but most other causes of oral pigmentation are uncommon or rare. Endocrinopathies (Addison's disease: Nelson's syndrome), drugs (e.g. antimalarials), naevi, and melanomas must all be considered in the differential diagnosis, as well as a range of other rare conditions.

(b) Weight loss, lassitude, weakness, anorexia, and hyperpigmentation — particularly of pigmented areas (nipples, genitalia), sun-exposed areas, and traumatized areas (e.g. skin flexures).

(c) Hypotension, hyperpigmentation, and reduced level of plasma cortisol and reduced cortisol secretion in response to injection of adrenocorticotrophic hormone (Synacthen test). Endogenous ACTH levels are raised in Addison's disease but reduced when hypoadrenocorticism is secondary to pituitary disease.

(d) Such surgical treatment may precipitate hypotensive collapse unless corticosteroids are given pre-operatively. This usually comprises 100–200 mg hydrocortisone hemisuccinate intravenously 30 minutes pre-operatively.

NB The patient included for comparison of skin colour has Paget's disease of bone in the left maxilla (Q1.2 (ii)).

A 1.3 (a) Angular cheilitis (angular stomatitis: perlèche). Erythema, fissuring, or, occasionally, ulceration is characteristic of angular cheilitis.

(b) (i) Inadequate dentures.
(ii) Chronic atrophic candidosis beneath a denture serves as a source of infection.
(iii) Xerostomia (leading to infection with candida).

(iv) Deficiencies of iron, folate, vitamin B12, or riboflavin. Most cases are related to (i) and (ii).

(c) Candida albicans, Staphylococcus aureus, streptoccocci.

(d) Investigate for underlying immunodeficiency, vitamin deficiency or Crohn's disease.

(e) (i) Instruct patient to leave the dentures out of mouth at night and stored in hypochlorite.
  (ii) Treat intraoral candidosis and angular cheilitis with antifungals (e.g. miconazole).
  (iii) Check the dentures for their adequacy.
  (iv) Consider the possibility of xerostomia or deficiency state.

A 1.4   (a) Cervical lymph node enlargement.

(b) (i) *History* directed particularly to elicit local lesions in the head and neck; fatigue or weight loss; or fever. Also, medical history considered with particular regard to tuberculosis and to previous lesions in the head and neck region.
  (ii) *Physical examination* directed particularly to elicit local lesions anywhere on the face, scalp, ears, mouth, sinus, pharynx, etc. Also, examination for enlarged lymph nodes elsewhere, such as in the axilla or inguinal region, and for enlarged liver and/or spleen. An ENT opinion may well be indicated — particularly to exclude a nasopharyngeal neoplasm.
  (iii) *Investigations* must be directed from the history and examination findings.

(c) Differential diagnosis
  Most enlarged lymph nodes in the neck are due to lymphadenitis caused by a viral upper respiratory tract infection but there are more serious causes to be considered.

  (i) *Inflammatory*
  Viral upper respiratory or oral infections
  Glandular fever syndromes (in younger patients)
  Cat scratch fever
  Specific bacterial infections: tuberculosis, syphilis, and atypical mycobacteria
  Non-specific bacterial infections: e.g. dental abscess, any local upper respiratory, oral or cutaneous infection
  Staphylococcal lymphadenitis (in childhood)
  Fungal infections RARELY: e.g. histoplasmosis
  Parasitic infestations: e.g. toxoplasmosis

    (ii) *Immunological*
      Some connective tissue disorders
      Acquired immune deficiency syndrome (AIDS) and the related persistent lymphadenopathy syndrome (PLS) (in young males)
      Sarcoidosis
    (iii) *Neoplastic*
      Malignant neoplasms in the head and neck; particularly oral, skin, upper respiratory, and thyroid
      Metastases from elsewhere: e.g. *occasionally* from gastric carcinoma
      Lymphoreticular neoplasms: leukaemia, lymphomas
    (iv) *Others*
      Some drugs: e.g. phenytoin

A 1.5   (a) Lack of zygomatic prominence.

      (b) Zygomatic hypoplasia *or* malunion of a fractured zygoma.

      (c) Many patients with this long-term deformity are not concerned about their appearance and no treatment is required. Surgical solutions include onlay grafts with autogenous bone or allografts, usually using carbon fibre materials such as Proplast. Local zygomatic osteotomies have been described, but morbidity tends to be high with these more complex procedures.

Examination of the face from above is an indispensable part of the examination both in cases of facial deformity and patients with a history of trauma to the maxillo-facial region. Zygomatic asymmetry is hard to detect from profile and full face examination.

Zygomatic hypoplasia is uncommon, but may be due to lack of growth as a result of embryological damage or damage at birth.

Classically, a fractured zygomatic complex involves fractures of the four sites where the zygomatic bone articulates with the rest of the facial skeleton, i.e. at the zygomatico-frontal, zygomatico-temporal and zygomatico-maxillary suture regions and at the lateral wall of the maxillary antrum.

A 1.6   (a) Herpetiform ulcers.

      (b) Minor aphthae and major aphthae. See A4.11

      (c) (i) Chlorhexidine (0.2 per cent aqueous mouthwash or 1 per cent gel).
        (ii) Corlan pellets (2.5 mg hydrocortisone hemisuccinate).
       (iii) Adcortyl in orabase (Triamcinolone acetonide).

(iv) Mysteclin capsules (tetracycline and amphotericin) one emptied into 5 ml water as a mouthwash may be useful in herpetiform ulcers;
plus many proprietary preparations often of doubtful value. More potent corticosteroids such as betamethasone may be effective but may also cause adrenal suppression.

There are multiple ovoid or round ulcers. These ulcers are termed herpetiform since the clinical appearance resembles acute herpetic stomatitis. However, unlike herpetic stomatitis, in patients with herpetiform ulcers there is no acute gingivitis, no fever or other systemic manifestations and the herpetiform ulcers are recurrent.

A 1.7   (a) Tetracycline staining.

(b) The patient may have had recurrent infections which necessitated tetracycline therapy. He may have, for example, cystic fibrosis or an immunodeficiency. This patient had had an immune defect since early childhood — the position of staining demonstrates exposure to tetracycline from this time.

(c) For improvement of aesthetics, veneers or crowns may be indicated.

The typical yellow, brown, and grey banded intrinsic staining in otherwise morphologically fairly normal teeth is indicative of tetracycline staining. These teeth fluoresce in ultra-violet light. Even short courses of tetracycline given to a pregnant mother or to a child under the age of 7 to 8 years may cause staining.

A 1.8   (a) Chronic haemorrhage from a gastro-intestinal lesion. Peptic ulcer, ulcerative colitis, or a neoplasm are among the common causes.

(b) Endoscopy; barium enema, barium meal and follow-through radiography; biopsy.

(c) (i) Coeliac disease (gluten-sensitive enteropathy).
   (ii) Crohn's disease.
   (iii) Ulcerative colitis.

In this patient multiple ulcers and polyps were revealed, predominantly in the sigmoid colon, suggestive of ulcerative colitis. This is pyostomatitis vegetans.

A 1.9   (a) Lichen planus.

(b) Dermatitis herpetiformis.

(c) Direct immunofluorescent tests on oral, or cutaneous biopsies, show granular deposits of IgA in the papillae of the lamina propria. A related disease — linear IgA disease — is characterized by linear deposits of IgA at the epithelial basement membrane zone (see A2.9).

(d) Dapsone (or sulphapyridine); often a gluten-free diet.

Oral lesions in dermatitis herpetiformis (DH) may be erythematous, vesicular, purpuric, or erosive although reports vary as to the prevalence of oral involvement.

DH is related to coeliac disease, and is characterized by a pruritic rash on extensor surfaces (see fig A1.9).

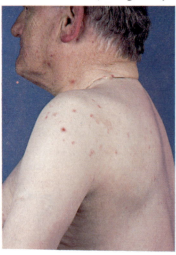

Fig. A1.9

A 1.10 (a) Glossitis (depapillation: bald tongue).

(b) Oral ulceration, oral candidosis (including angular cheilitis), and glossitis are features of deficiency of iron, folic acid, or vitamin B12.

(c) These are spoon-shaped nails (koilonychia) suggestive of iron deficiency.

(d) In iron deficiency a full blood picture (microcytosis), red cell indices (reduced MCV, MCH and possibly MCHC), and iron studies (low serum ferritin) are most useful. Remember to establish the *cause* of the deficiency, which is usually chronic haemorrhage from the genito-urinary or gastrointestinal tract. This patient proved to have gastric carcinoma.

The tongue is depapillated and red as well as having a scrotal appearance. Depapillation is usually caused by a deficiency state, but may be seen in other conditions such as lichen planus, vesiculobullous disorders, or Sjögren's syndrome.

A 1.11 (a) This was a misdiagnosis. These are Fordyce spots (ectopic sebaceous glands). These are also common in the buccal mucosa as a yellowish small granular rash.

(b) Sebaceous glands.

(c) No treatment, except reassurance, is needed.

A 1.12 (a) (i) Local tumour — particularly a carcinoma.
(ii) Metastatic carcinoma from the lung.
(iii) Tuberculosis.
This proved to be a secondary deposit from bronchogenic carcinoma in a patient with carcinomatosis.

(b) (i) Oral examination, radiography and biopsy.
(ii) General examination, chest radiography, and probably a skeletal radiographic survey and/or bone scan.

Metastasis to the oral tissues from distant neoplasms is uncommon but carcinomas of bronchus, breast, stomach, thyroid, and kidney may metastasize — particularly to the mandibular premolar region.

A 1.13 (a) (i) Airway control. The injury described will involve the musculature of the tongue and soft palate. It is likely that, following such a midline injury, there will be detachment of all genial muscles and probably hypoglossal nerve paraesis and anaesthesia of the tongue. This particular patient had also in fact sustained a midline fracture of the mandible. The mouth and pharynx must be cleared of debris, broken teeth, dentures, blood, etc. In an unconscious patient, an airway should be inserted as soon as possible and also a towel-clip or suture inserted anteriorly into the tongue and traction applied to pull the tongue anteriorly. The patient should be placed in the tonsillar (head injury) position so that gravity will take blood etc. out of the mouth rather than into the pharynx.
(ii) Control of haemorrhage is performed by applying pressure with 4 in. × 4 in. gauze or ribbon gauze. If bleeding

continues to be a problem the patient should be taken to the operating theatre for identification of bleeding points and suturing and for nasal packing if necessary. Definitive closure of lacerations, and reduction and fixation of fractures may then be undertaken.

(b) Low velocity wounds are characterized by entrance and exit wounds of approximately the same size, with only a narrow tract of non-vital tissue between. Low velocity projectiles will be deflected by structures such as the mandible and teeth and, commonly, the projectile is retained in the tissues. High velocity injuries are characterized by a small entrance wound and a very much larger exit wound. Between the two a cone-shaped cavity of tissue is rendered non-vital by the high pressure wave preceding, and vacuum following, the projectile as it passes through the tissues. Deflection of projectiles is usually uncommon and disintegration of the skeleton is the norm. The partial vacuum following the projectile will attract foreign bodies such as pieces of clothing and also fragments of bone and teeth. These commonly increase the risk of supervening infection. In contrast with low velocity injuries, high velocity wounds normally involve substantial tissue loss and definitive treatment may therefore necessitate grafting of soft tissue and bone.

A 1.14 (a) Occipito-mental view. This is an extremely useful view in the investigation of any condition affecting the middle third of the facial skeleton, including traumatic conditions. The base of the skull which would overlie the facial skeleton in a standard postero-anterior view, is effectively excluded.

(b) 1. Fracture of left infraorbital margin.
2. Fracture affecting the body of the left zygoma.
3. Fracture affecting the lateral wall of left maxillary antrum.
4. Fracture involving left fronto-zygomatic suture region.
5. Diminution in the size of the maxillary antrum.
6. Opacity of the left maxillary antrum.
7. Superimposition of the left zygomatic body on the coronoid process.

(c) Fractured zygomatic complex. This is one of the most common maxillo-facial fractures, often caused by inter-personal violence, trauma during sport, road traffic accidents, etc.

This view is inadequate in the examination of the zygomatic *arch* and a submentovertical view may provide more information. This occipito-mental view is obtained by passing X-rays infra-superiorly and bone displacement in the antero-posterior plane is therefore most evident. Displacement is not always in this plane and a second occipito-mental radiograph with X-rays passing in a more antero-posterior plane may demonstrate infra-superior displacement.

A 1.15 (a) Xerostomia: probably because of Sjögren's syndrome

(b) There is no specific blood test to diagnose Sjögren's syndrome but the following findings are typical.
  (i) Raised erythrocyte sedimentation rate (or plasma viscosity).
  (ii) Rheumatoid factor or other auto-antibodies (particularly anti-SSA and anti-SSB).
  (iii) Hypergammaglobulinaemia.

(c) The main complications of severe persistent xerostomia apart from oral discomfort include susceptibility to
  (i) Disturbed taste sensation.
  (ii) Candidosis.
  (iii) Caries.
  (iv) Periodontal disease.
  (v) Ascending sialadenitis.
  (iv) Difficulties in denture retention, speaking, and swallowing.

The tongue is very dry and slightly lobulated and depapillated.

The complaint of dry mouth is common and usually is related to the use of drugs with atropine like activity (e.g. tricyclic antidepressants), or to sympathomimetic drugs. On the other hand, depressed patients may complain of a dry mouth *per se* and this is by no means always confirmed by examination of salivary function.

Organic disease of the salivary glands may cause xerostomia as in this patient who also had dry eyes (xerophthalmia) and rheumatoid arthritis (the illustration shows rheumatoid nodules). The triad of xerostomia, xerophthalmia, and a connective tissue disorder (usually rheumatoid arthritis) is termed Sjögren's syndrome (sometimes called *secondary* Sjögren's syndrome). A less common variant in which patients do *not* have a connective tissue disorder, is the Sicca syndrome (sometimes termed *primary* Sjögren's syndrome).

The illustrations overleaf show the hands in rheumatoid arthritis with typical ulnar deviation of the fingers (fig A1.15(i)), and a normal parotid sialogram together with one showing sialectasis in Sjögren's syndrome (fig A1.15(ii)).

Other organic causes of xerostomia include irradiation damage of the major salivary glands, and severe dehydration.

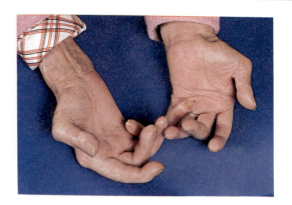

Fig. A1.15(i)

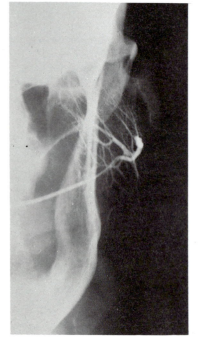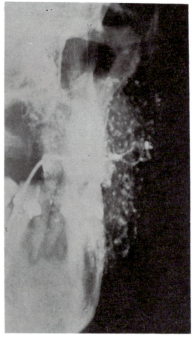

Fig. A1.15(ii)

PAPER 2

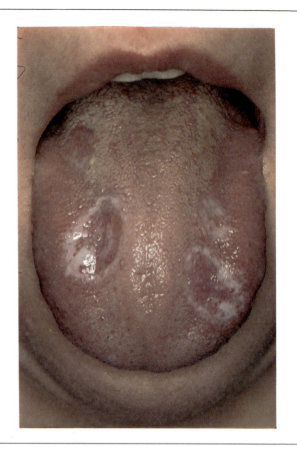

Q 2.1 (a) This patient complained of a chronically sore tongue. What is the probable cause?

(b) How would you establish the diagnosis?

(c) How might you manage this patient?

(d) What, if any, systemic disorders may be associated?

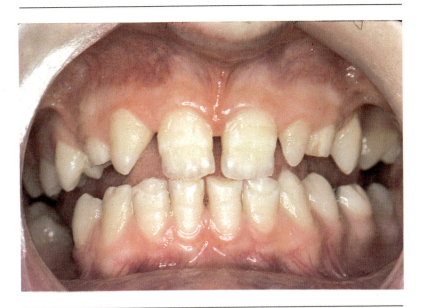

Q 2.2 This is a young adult who complained of poor aesthetics from the
age of 9 years when the incisors appeared.

(a) $\lfloor 2$ is peg-shaped and $\underline{C}|\underline{C}$ are retained. Why is $\underline{C}\rfloor$ retained?

(b) During what period of life has odontogenesis been disturbed?

(c) This patient was blind, from cataracts, and was 4 ft. 6 in. in
height. What single diagnosis would explain all these features?

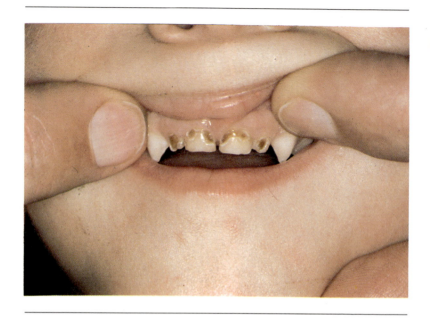

Q 2.3   (a) Are these deciduous or permanent teeth?

(b) What is the cause of the brown lesions?

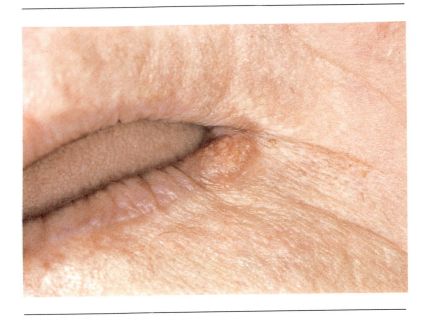

Q 2.4   This lady noticed a small persistent lump on her lower lip.

(a) What is the probable diagnosis?

(b) What investigation(s), if any, is/are necessary?

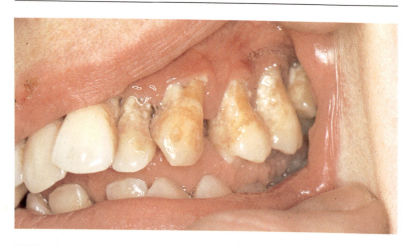

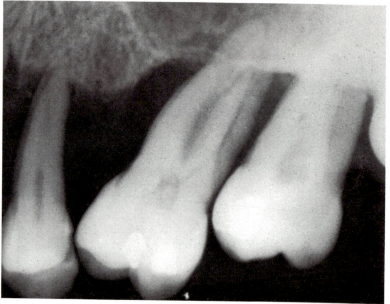

Q 2.5 This 32 year old female complained of loose teeth.

(a) What comments would you make on her periodontal state.

(b) What disorder(s) should be excluded?

(c) What other lesion (of microbial aetiology) is present?

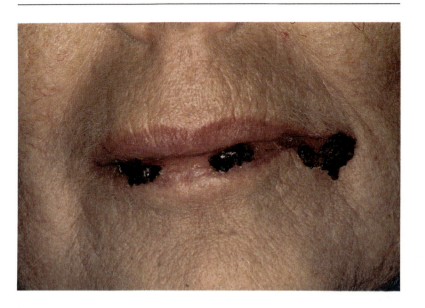

Q 2.6 (a) This is a 60 year old female in-patient with leukaemia. What are
these lesions?

(b) How would you establish the diagnosis?

(c) How could you manage this patient's oral lesions?

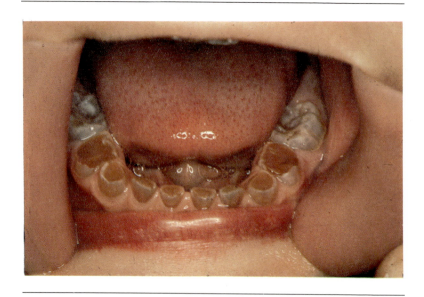

Q 2.7   (a) What is the diagnosis?

(b) What other problems may be present?

(c) What treatment is indicated?

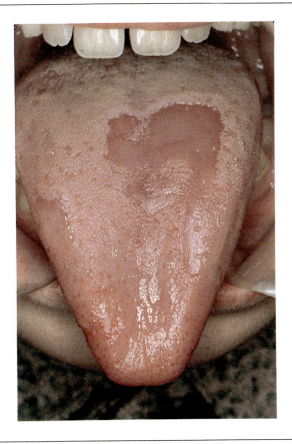

Q 2.8 (a) This patient complained of a sore tongue. What is the probable
                diagnosis?

         (b) Can this be associated with any other condition?

         (c) What is the treatment?

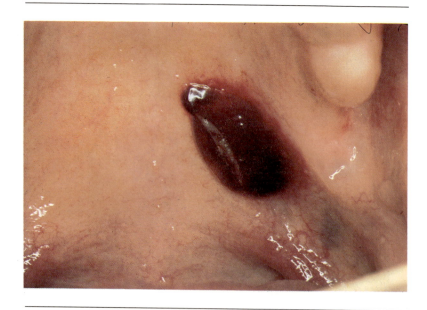

Q 2.9 (a) What is the palatal lesion shown here?

(b) What is the differential diagnosis?

(c) How is the diagnosis established?

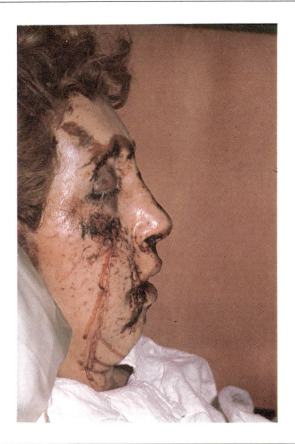

Q 2.10 This 18 year old man was involved in a road traffic accident.

   (a) Which five abnormalities seen here may be features of fractures of the facial skeleton?

   (b) In the absence of intra-cranial injury which cranial nerves may be damaged and which functions of these nerves should there-fore be particularly examined?

   (c) Which categories of fixation would be utilized here?

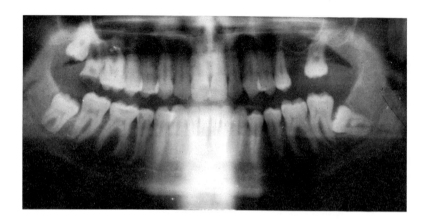

Q 2.11 This panoramic radiograph was taken of a 27 year old man complaining of all the symptoms of pulpitis associated with 7⌋. Apart from caries of this and other teeth and some mild gingivitis there were no other abnormalities clinically. There is no history of pericoronitis.

(a) What abnormalities are shown on this radiograph?

(b) If extraction of lower third molars is contemplated under local anaesthesia from which site should bone be removed?

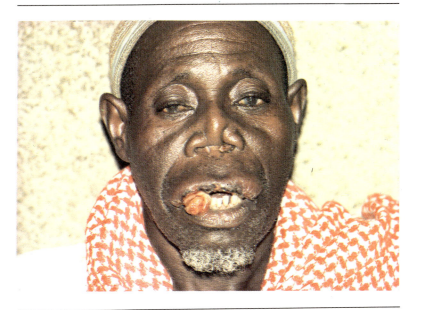

Q 2.12 This man presented in a Nigerian Oral Surgery Department with granulomatous lesions affecting the mouth and lips together with apparent destruction of the nasal septum.

(a) What is the probable diagnosis?

(b) List the other clinical features of this condition.

(c) What is the causative factor and how may it be identified?

(d) What is the treatment?

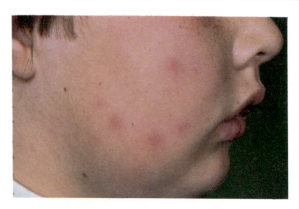

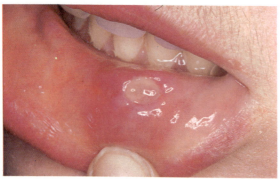

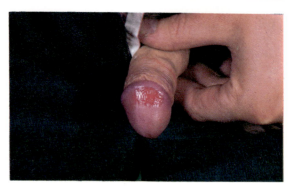

Q 2.13 (a) What is the differential diagnosis?

(b) What is the common 'serious' visual complication?

(c) How do the oral ulcers shown here differ from aphthous ulcers?

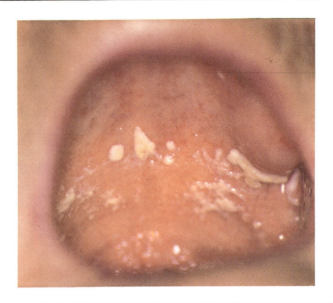

Q 2.14 (a) This bedridden geriatric patient complained of a sore palate. What is the probable diagnosis?

      (b) How might you establish the diagnosis?

      (c) Are any other investigations needed?

      (d) How would you manage the patient?

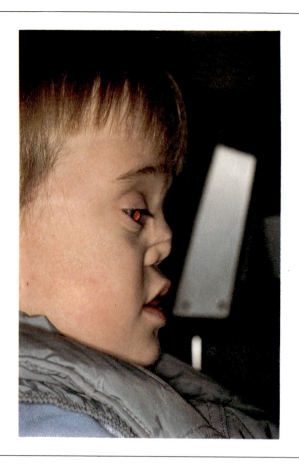

Q 2.15 (a) Which abnormalities are seen here?

(b) Of which broad category of cranio-facial disorders is this an example?

A 2.1 (a) Lichen planus.

(b) (i) Examination for lesions elsewhere in the mouth, particularly in the buccal mucosa and on the skin.

(ii) Biopsy (see also A2.9).

(c) Topical corticosteroids (see also A1.6).

(d) Lichen planus is usually *NOT* associated with systemic disease. Occasional associations may include:
Diabetes mellitus
Hypertension
Ulcerative colitis
Primary biliary cirrhosis
Chronic active hepatitis
Graft-versus-host disease
Immunodeficiency
Autoimmune disorders such as lupus erythematosus or pemphigoid
Drugs, particularly antidiabetics, antihypertensives, anti-inflammatory non-steroidal agents, and antimalarials.

The circinate white lesions are fairly typical of lichen planus, although lichen planus may also present with papules, plaques, or striae. The appearance in this patient might be confused with erythema migrans but in the latter the margins of the lesions are yellowish and the centre usually depapillated while the position and the shape of lesions constantly changes (see A2.8 and A3.1).

Topical corticosteroids, particularly hydrocortisone hemisuccinate pellets or triamcinolone acetonide in orabase are the most commonly effective agents. Many other drugs, such as etretinate, griseofulvin, etc., have been tried but the adverse reactions or doubtful efficacy tend to diminish their use in practice.

A 2.2 (a) Probably because 3| has erupted mesially into 2| space. C| roots have therefore not been resorbed.

(b) In infancy: the crowns of the incisors, which are forming at that time, are malformed (hypoplastic).

(c) Idiopathic hypoparathyroidism.

Delayed eruption, enamel hypoplasia, cataracts, and short stature can all be explained by hypoparathyroidism. The missing teeth may be co-incidental.

Other features of idiopathic hypoparathyroidism may include epilepsy, tetany, mental handicap, chronic mucocutaneous candidosis, and polyendocrinopathies.

A 2.3   (a) Deciduous teeth.

(b) Dental caries.

Deciduous teeth erupt after about the age of 6 months and their permanent successors appear in the mouth after the age of about 6–7 years, though it may be a further 6 years before the majority have erupted.

Dental bacterial plaque metabolizes refined carbohydrates (mainly sucrose) to organic acids, which decalcify the enamel. The early lesion is white but eventually the caries breaks through into dentine and advances rapidly, becoming brown as shown. Eventually the tooth dies and may become abscessed, or the crown breaks away as shown here. If the area becomes 'self-cleansing' caries may be arrested and appear as dark brown eburnated dentine (Fig. A2.3).

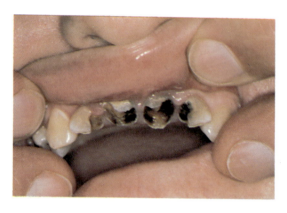

Fig. A2.3

A 2.4   (a) Squamous cell carcinoma.

(b) Biopsy.

Squamous carcinoma affects the lower lip predominantly and is a disease mainly of caucasians, particularly elderly males who work outdoors or who have extensive exposure to sunlight. Occasionally, keratoacanthoma or basal cell carcinoma appear on the lower lip.

Any lump persisting for more than three weeks should be biopsied. The prognosis for labial carcinoma is excellent, with more than 75–85 per cent 5 year survival. The earlier the diagnosis, the better the prognosis and the better the aesthetic results of treatment.

A 2.5 (a) The oral hygiene is poor but, even so, the periodontal destruction far exceeds that which would under normal circumstances be present at this age. This rapidly destructive periodontitis suggests an abnormal host response to dental bacterial plaque.

(b) (i) Diabetes mellitus (which was the diagnosis here)
(ii) Leucocyte or other immune disorders (including Down's syndrome).
(iii) Rapidly progressive periodontitis.

(c) Recurrent herpes labialis (cold sore).

A 2.6 (a) Herpes labialis.

(b) Viral swabs of the lesions sent, in viral transport medium, for culture of herpes simplex virus on baby hamster kidney (BHK) cells, *OR* electron microscopy, if vesicle fluid is available. Serology is of little value in this instance.

(c) With topical 5 per cent idoxuridine, or 5 per cent acyclovir cream, *OR* if there are extending lesions and the threat of systematization, treatment may need to be systemic acyclovir, inosine, or vidarabine.

Haemorrhagic crusts on the vermilion and at the mucocutaneous junction are caused by bleeding into the lesion as a consequence of the thrombocytopenia of leukaemia. Recurrent herpetic lesions usually affect mucocutaneous junctions but, in the immuno-compromised (such as leukaemia or AIDS,) oral lesions may occur — as severe spreading dendritic ulcers.

A 2.7 (a) Dentinogenesis imperfecta.

(b) Osteogenesis imperfecta (fractures), deafness, etc. (see A3.8).

(c) The softness of the dentine impairs the life of restorations so that full coverage crowns may be needed to improve aesthetics in teenagers.

This is the primary dentition. The teeth may be translucent brown or purplish in colour. Although the enamel is normal, the dentine is abnormal leading to weakness at the amelodentinal junction such that the enamel is shed under the trauma of mastication, leading to attrition as shown. Obliteration of the pulp by dentine usually prevents traumatic exposure.

The amelodentinal junction loses its scalloping, the dentine consists of irregular tubules and roots are short, blunted and susceptible to fractures.

Radiographs show obliteration, partially or totally, of the pulp chamber and root canals which is virtually pathognomonic (Fig A2.7).

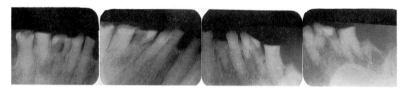

Fig. A2.7

A 2.8 (a) Geographic tongue.

(b) Fissured tongue.

(c) Erythema migrans is a benign disorder for which there is no known treatment.

The patches of depapillation on the tongue are characteristic of geographic tongue (erythema migrans; benign migratory glossitis) and the history almost invariably confirms the appearance of red patches that increase in size and change in shape before healing, and affect different sites on the tongue. Erythema migrans rarely affects the labial, buccal, or palatal mucosa.

The aetiology of this common condition is unknown and there are no associations with serious disorders. There *may* be an association with atopic disorders.

Lingual depapillation is also seen in deficiency states (of iron, folic acid, vitamin B_{12} etc.) and in ulcerative conditions.

Although erythema migrans often occurs in the absence of a fissured tongue, patients with the latter often have the former.

A 2.9 (a) A blood-filled bulla.

(b) Pemphigoid (mucous membrane or cicatricial) or angina bullosa haemorrhagica are the most likely diagnoses, but pemphigus and a bleeding disorder must be excluded.

(c) (i) History, examination.
(ii) Investigations if necessary to exclude a bleeding tendency (see A5.10).

(iii) Biopsy of the lesion examined histologically and by direct immunofluorescence (IF). In pemphigoid there is sub-epithelial vesiculation and deposits of C3 and often IgG at the epithelial basement membrane zone (see Fig. A2.9(i)). In pemphigus, deposits of IgG are found mainly inter-cellularly in the stratum spinosum (Fig. A2.9(ii)): acan-tholysis leads to intra-epithelial vesiculation.

(iv) Serum, for autoantibodies to epithelial constituents deter-mined by indirect immunofluorescence. In pemphigus there are autoantibodies to epithelial inter-cellular cement. In some patients with pemphigoid there are circulating anti-bodies directed against the basement membrane zone.

NB   Direct IF is particularly valuable in the diagnosis of pemphigus and is also valuable in pemphigoid, dermatitis herpetiformis, and linear IgA disease (see A1.9). Direct IF is of little value in the diagnosis of erythema multiforme (see A4.9). In lichen planus direct IF findings are non-specific but may help differentiation from lupus erythematosus (see A1.9, A2.1, A5.15, and Table A2.9).

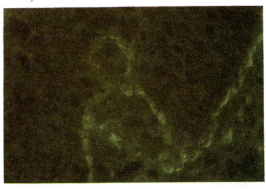

Pemphigoid

Fig. A2.9(i)

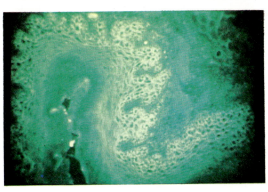

Pemphigus

Fig. A2.9(ii)

Table A2.9

Disease	DIF*	Deposits	Pattern of IF	IIF**	Autoantibodies
Pemphigus	+	IgG C3	epithelial inter-cellular	+	epithelial inter-cellular
Mucous membrane pemphigoid	+	C3 IgG	linear epithelial basement membrane zone	±	none or epithelial basement membrane
Bullous pemphigoid	+	IgG C3	linear epithelial basement membrane zone	+	epithelial basement membrane
Dermatitis herpetiformis	+	IgA C3	linear or fibrillar epithelial basement membrane zone	–	gliaden and/or reticulin
Erythema multiforme	+	C3 IgM	vessel walls in lamina propria	–	–
Lichen planus	±	IgM, IgG, IgA C3	globular epithelial or lamina propria	–	–
Discoid lupus erythematosus	+	IgA, IgG, IgM C3	granular epithelial basement membrane zone	±	none or antinuclear

*DIF = direct immunofluorescence   **IIF = indirect immunofluorescence

A 2.10 (a) (i) Periorbital haematoma.
  (ii) Elongation of the face.
  (iii) Facial swelling.
  (iv) Anterior open bite.
  (v) Epistaxis.

(b) An examination of such a patient should always include an assessment of the function of all cranial nerves if possible. Assuming a Le Fort III fracture and a fractured mandible, then the following neurological abnormalities are possible:
  I.   Olfactory nerve. Anosmia due to a fracture of the cribriform plate. This is nearly always impossible to assess due to nasal obstruction by blood clots during the early phase.
  II. Optic nerve. Visual acuity is sometimes impaired due to orbital apex bleeding, but this is rare.
  III. Oculomotor nerve. This nerve supplies all the extraocular muscles except lateral rectus and superior oblique. It also supplies levator palpebrae superioris and constrictor

pupillae. Ophthalmoplegia is sometimes a feature of the supraorbital fissure syndrome where the fissure has been collapsed. In the absence of superior orbital fissure damage, third cranial nerve injury is rare.

IV. Trochlear nerve. Superior oblique muscle palsy is rare after trauma.

V. Trigeminal nerve.
   (i) Ophthalmic division. Frontal hypoaesthesia may be a feature of superior orbital fissure syndrome when supraorbital and/or supratrochlear nerves have been damaged.
   (ii) Maxillary division. Infraorbital hypoaesthesia follows infraorbital trauma and hypoaesthesia of the upper teeth may follow posterior superior dental, middle superior dental, and anterior superior dental nerve damage. Zygomatico-temporal and zygomatico-facial nerve function may be impaired in patients with zygomatic trauma.
   (iii) Mandibular division. Mental hypoaesthesia and hypoaesthesia affecting the mandibular teeth and attached mucosa may follow inferior dental nerve damage. Auriculotemporal nerve damage results occasionally in scalp hypoaesthesia. Occasionally fractures at the angle of the mandible result in lingual nerve hypoaesthesia, or mylohyoid nerve damage, resulting in submental hypoaesthesia.

VI. Abducent nerve. This nerve supplies lateral rectus. Lateral rectus palsy is sometimes a feature of fractures of the lateral orbital wall.

VII. Facial nerve. Facial lacerations are most often responsible for paralysis of the muscles of facial expression in trauma cases. Branches passing over the zygoma may occasionally be damaged and impair the function of frontalis muscle and sphincteric muscles around the eyes, nose, and mouth. Occasionally the facial nerve is damaged by impaction of the ascending ramus of the mandible against the mastoid process and a total lower motor nerve injury may then be apparent.

VIII.–XI. Not usually involved.

XII. Not usually involved, except in extensive lacerations of the tongue.

(c) Cranio-maxillary or cranio-mandibular fixation.

The occlusion is not shown by this photograph, but the lips apart position seen is very often indicative of posterior gagging of the occlusion.

Le Fort described three common sites for middle third facial fractures:
1. Low level type I where the hard palate and tooth-bearing alveolus is detached from the remainder of the facial skeleton.
2. Pyramidal type II where a pyramidal-shaped fragment is detached, involving the nasal bones, and sometimes extending into the cribriform plate. (This is the most common type)
3. High level type III where all the bones of the facial skeleton are detached from the skull base.

A 2.11 (a) Impacted $\overline{8|8}$ and unerupted $\underline{8|}$ with caries $\underline{7|}$ and $\overline{65|}$.

(b) Buccal bone should be removed to create a mesial application point and to clear the buccal aspect of the crown. The $8|$ may be disimpacted either by dividing the tooth vertically or by removing distal bone. The curvature of the mesial root will probably necessitate root division anyway. The same technique applies to the $\lceil 8$ although distal bone removal will certainly be required for disimpaction (unless the lingual split technique is used).

The mere presence of impacted third molars is no indication for removal. Pericoronitis is rare after the age of 25, as is follicular (dentigerous) cyst development. These third molars are unlikely to influence incisor position at this age. Removal may, in fact, be easier later due to the slow eruption which may accompany mesial drift secondary to interproximal wear or, in this case, to the extraction of other teeth for any reason. However, surgery in general is less hazardous in the younger patient.

A 2.12 (a) Lepromatous leprosy.

(b) Other clinical features include widespread lesions affecting the skin, sometimes preceded by a rash of the macular or papular type. The neural form of leprosy is characterized by loss of sensory function particularly with regard to pain and touch. Classically, leprosy causes thickening of the greater auricular nerve, visible in the neck.

(c) Mycobacterium leprae. This may be identified from a smear of the fluid from a skin lesion stained with Ziehl–Neelsen stain. Histological examination of a biopsied skin lesion will reveal bundles of red leprosy bacilli inside mononuclear cells (tissue stained with Triff stain).

(d) The management of leprosy is largely using the sulfone group of drugs (Dapsone). Streptomycin may also be used.
Oral manifestations of leprosy may comprise gingival en-

largements and tooth mobility, ulceration, and exophytic granulomatous lesions which can affect the tongue, lips, or hard
palate and nasal septum. Leprosy occasionally is seen in the
U.K. in immigrants.

NB Although rarely seen in Western Europe and North America, it has
been estimated that there are approximately 5 million people with leprosy in
the world today. The important differential diagnosis is from syphilis, yaws,
tuberculosis of the skin, ringworm, and neuritis.

A 2.13 (a) (i) Behcet's syndrome.
          (ii) Ulcerative colitis.

        (b) Ocular disease (uveitis) may be found in Behcet's syndrome or
            ulcerative colitis.

        (c) They do not.

Oral and genital ulcers with cutaneous lesions may be found in Behcet's
syndrome, erythema multiforme, lichen planus, pemphigus, pemphigoid
ulcerative colitis, syphilis, and some vitamin deficiency states. Oral ulcers are
associated with urethritis and conjunctivitis in Reiter's syndrome.

Behcet's syndrome is a rare disease characterized by aphthous oral ulcers,
genital ulcers, and uveitis. A multi-system disorder, it may be complicated by
arthritic symptoms or by cutaneous, vascular, neurological, or other lesions.

There is no specific diagnostic test. Venepuncture occasionally is followed
by pustule formation. Various immunological abnormalities may be found,
particularly high levels of circulating immune complexes. An immune
complex aetiology is suggested by the clinical features of arthralgia, fever,
and rashes such as erythema nodosum (see Fig. A2.13). HLA-typing may

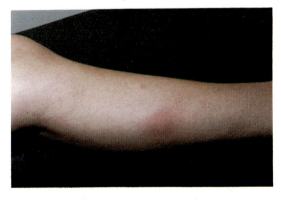

Fig. A2.13

offer some guidance particularly as to whether manifestations are most likely to involve the eyes (HLA-B5) or joints (HLA-B27).

A 2.14 (a) Thrush (acute pseudomembranous candidosis).

(b) (i) Lesions wipe off with gauze.
(ii) Swab shows hyphae of candida species.
(iii) Culture.

(c) Exclude local causes such as antimicrobial or corticosteroid therapy, underlying disease such as diabetes mellitus, immune defect or xerostomia from any cause. Thrush is a 'disease of the diseased'. (Remember that, in a younger patient, thrush is an early manifestation of AIDS.)

(d) Treat the underlying cause where possible. Antimycotic agents such as nystatin, 500 000 unit tablets or 100 000 unit pastilles q.d.s. or amphotericin 10 mg lozenges q.d.s. used for 2 to 4 weeks are indicated.

Thrush characteristically presents with this appearance 'similar to milk curds' and usually affects the palate and upper buccal vestibule. The underlying and adjacent mucosa may well be erythematous and sore.

Candida species, particularly *C. albicans* are common oral commensals. In some studies up to 50 per cent of the population have been demonstrated to be carriers of yeast forms of *C. albicans*. Candida colonises particularly the posterior dorsum of the tongue.

Candidosis is associated with the appearance of hyphal (mycelial) forms and may be acute or chronic, viz.

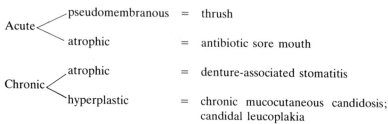

Acute — pseudomembranous = thrush
atrophic = antibiotic sore mouth

Chronic — atrophic = denture-associated stomatitis
hyperplastic = chronic mucocutaneous candidosis; candidal leucoplakia

A 2.15 (a) Proptosis, maxillary retrusion and nasal deformity.

(b) Both Apert's and Crouzon's syndromes are examples of craniosynostoses, or premature fusion of calvarial sutures. In Apert's syndrome the skull often assumes a deformity known as turribrachycephaly.

The other major facial characteristic of both Apert's and Crouzon's syndromes, (this is an example of Apert's syndrome) is hypertelorism. Apert's syndrome is characterized by the presence of syndactyly affecting both hands and feet and a general absence of inheritance. Crouzon's syndrome is strongly autosomal dominant however, and apart from occasional examples of elbow ankylosis and radius subluxation, this syndrome does not involve abnormalities in regions other than cranium and face.

PAPER 3

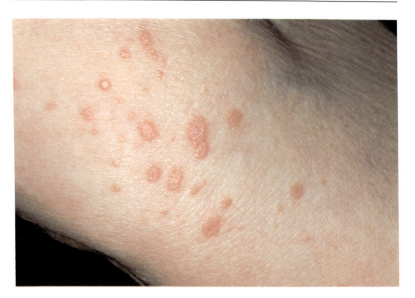

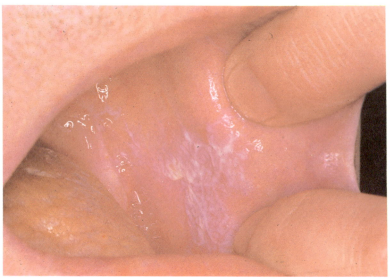

Q 3.1 (a) These illustrations are from the same patient. What is the diagnosis?

(b) What other forms can the oral lesions take?

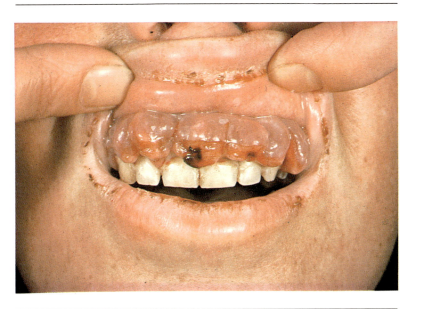

Q 3.2 This patient complained of severe persistent gingival haemorrhage over the previous 2 years.

(a) What is the most *common* cause of gingival haemorrhage?

(b) If associated with propensity to bruising, as in this patient, what disorders should be excluded?

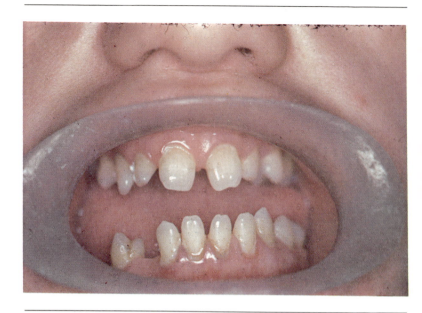

Q 3.3 (a) The appearance of these permanent teeth is fairly characteristic of which congenital disorder?

(b) What acquired disorder might cause hypoplasia in the *deciduous* dentition?

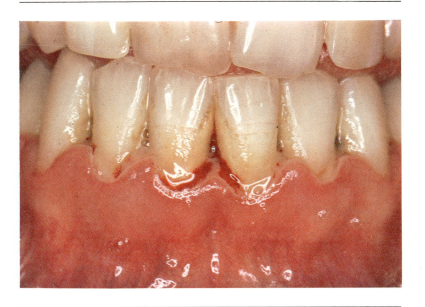

Q 3.4 This was a student who returned from a trip to India complaining of bleeding gums.

(a) What is the diagnosis?

(b) What is the treatment?

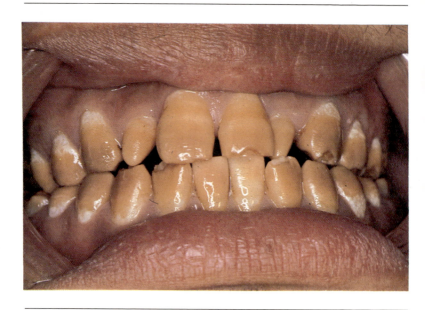

Q 3.5 This patient complained about the appearance of the teeth.

(a) What aspects of the history are important in establishing the diagnosis?

(b) What is the probable diagnosis?

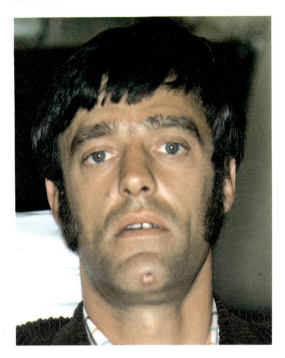

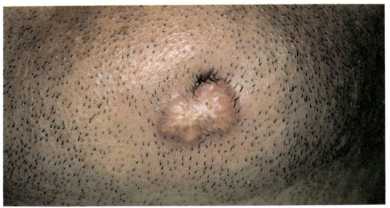

Q 3.6   This man complained of a persistent lump on his chin.

    (a) What is the differential diagnosis?

    (b) What is the most likely cause if the lesion is of dental origin?

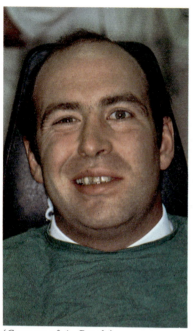 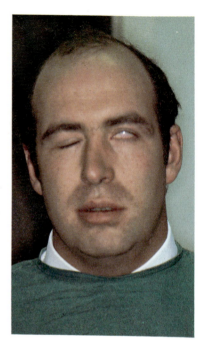

(*Courtesy of A. Brooks*)

Q 3.7   (a) What is the problem here?

(b) How would you localize the site of the lesion?

(c) What other complications may be present?

(d) If the patient presented shortly after the onset, how might you manage the problem?

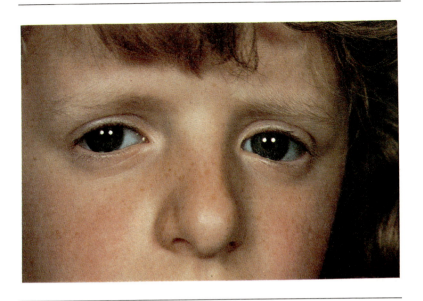

Q 3.8   (a)   What is shown here?

         (b)   What may be the oral complications?

         (c)   What other handicaps may be present?

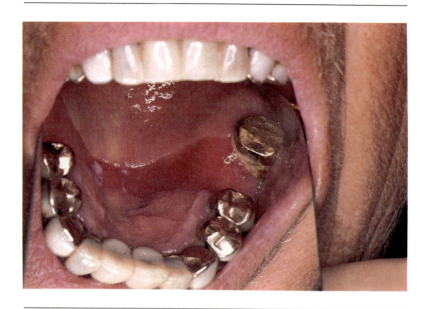

Q 3.9 (a) What is this condition?

(b) How would you manage the patient?

(c) What lesion may be associated with this condition?

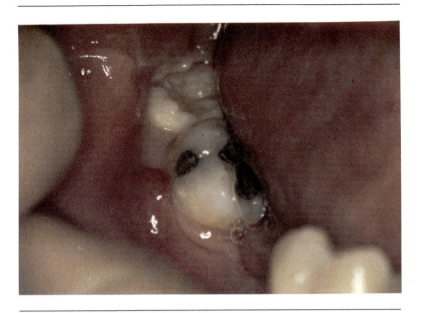

Q 3.10 (a) What two abnormalities are shown here?

(b) Explain how these two lesions can be part of the same pathologic process.

(c) What is the treatment?

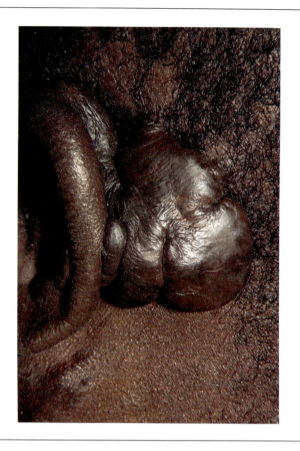

Q 3.11 (a) What is this lesion?

(b) Of what is it principally composed?

(c) Name four possible methods of treatment.

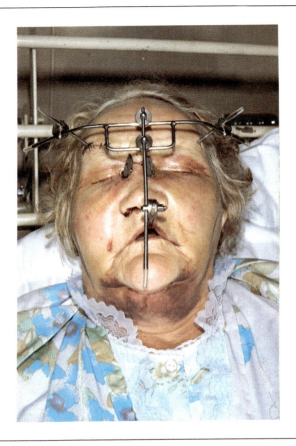

Q 3.12 This 74 year old lady was treated for a Le Fort II fracture and fractured nasal bones.

    (a) (i) Relating to the fractured maxilla, which category of fixation is employed here?

      (ii) What particular apparatus has been used?

    (b) What type of fixation has been applied to the fractured nasal bones?

    (c) What alternative methods are available for the fixation of fractured nasal bones?

    (d) To what structures are the medial canthal ligaments attached medially?

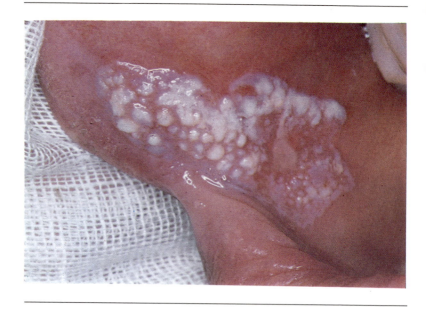

Q 3.13 (a) What is this lesion?

(b) What is the prognosis?

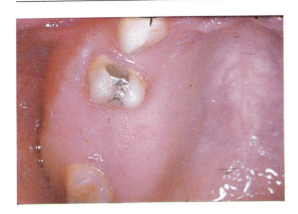

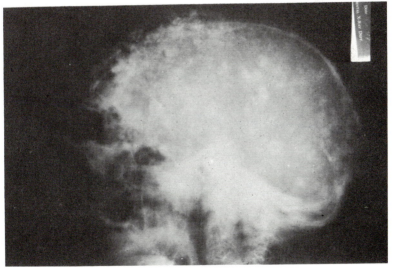

Q 3.14 This patient was referred with a hard swelling in the maxilla and complained of severe headaches. A clinical slide and skull radiograph are shown.

(a) What is the diagnosis?

(b) What are the oral complications?

(c) What blood tests may be useful in diagnosis?

(d) What is the treatment?

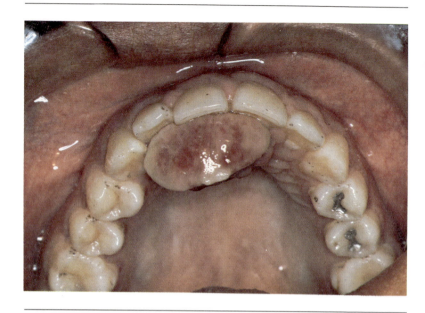

Q 3.15 This slide shows a gingival swelling in a 25-week pregnant patient.

(a) What is the cause?

(b) What is the treatment?

(c) Is this a common site for this particular lesion?

A 3.1   (a) Lichen planus.

(b) Papules, plaques, striae, erosions, or reticular as here. Bullae are rare.

Lichen planus characteristically causes bilateral reticular white lesions in the buccal mucosa and may produce a papular rash, especially on the wrists, as shown here (see also A2.1).

A 3.2   (a) Inflammatory periodontal disease (chronic gingivitis, acute gingivitis, and chronic periodontitis).

(b) A bleeding tendency such as is associated with a platelet defect or deficiency (e.g. leukaemia) must be excluded. This patient had vitamin C deficiency (scurvy) — a *rare* cause of gingival bleeding in the U.K.

Accumulation of dental bacterial plaque leads to inflammation, with hyperaemia and ulceration in the gingival sulcular epithelium, together with a tendency to bleed on minimal pressure such as toothbrushing.

A 3.3   (a) Congenital syphilis.

(b) Congenital rubella.

These are Hutchinson's teeth, which have a 'screwdriver' shape, sometimes with a notched incisal edge.
    Treponema pallidum appears only to infect the foetus after about the fifth month of intrauterine life and causes dental anomalies apparently because it affects the developing tooth germs.
    Hutchinson's triad is the teeth, interstitial keratitis and deafness. Patients may also be mentally handicapped.

A 3.4   (a) Acute ulcerative gingivitis (acute necrotising gingivitis; Vincent's disease; trench mouth).

(b) (i) Improved oral hygiene.
       (ii) Antimicrobials — metronidazole (or penicillin).
       (iii) Referral for periodontal care.

This is related to a fusospirochaetal infection but there is no evidence that it is contagious. The disease appears to be predisposed to by poor oral hygiene, smoking, 'stress', and viral respiratory infections.

Predominantly a disease of young adults, particularly those living in communities, acute ulcerative gingivitis is characterized by profuse gingival haemorrhage on the slightest pressure, soreness, halitosis, and unpleasant taste. The disease causes ulceration and destruction of the interdental papilla which appear blunted. Complications are rare in the U.K. although recurrence is fairly common (see also Cancrum Oris A4.6).

A 3.5   (a) (i) Family history — may be positive in amelogenesis imperfecta.

        (ii) Drug history — particularly of tetracycline use in the first 8 years of life.

        (iii) Origin of patient — particularly to exclude fluorosis.

        (iv) Whether the deciduous dentition was affected.

  (b) Amelogenesis imperfecta.

The enamel is dull brown and the disease affects all teeth equally as opposed to tetracycline staining which usually is more prominent anteriorly and may be 'banded'. Clearly the enamel is friable and has chipped away from at least $\dfrac{\mid 1\,3\,4\,5}{2\mid\ 2}$. Radiographs showed little enamel, further confirming the diagnosis.

NB The peg-shaped $2\mid2$ are irrelevant to this condition.

A 3.6   (a) (i) Cutaneous infection.

        (ii) Keloid scar.

        (iii) Dental infection discharging onto skin.

  (b) A chronic periapical abscess related to a lower incisor tooth that has become non-vital through caries or trauma. Physicians often overlook the dental origin of such lesions overlying the mandible or in the submental or submandibular regions (see Fig. A3.6).

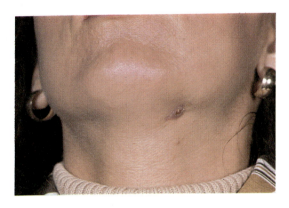

Fig. A3.6

A 3.7   (a) Unilateral facial palsy on the left side (Bell's palsy in this patient).

(b) A lower motor neurone lesion of the facial nerve, e.g. Bell's palsy, paralyses one side of the face completely. Some movement of the forehead is retained in an upper motor neurone lesion such as a stroke (as are involuntary movements, for example, facial movements when laughing spontaneously).

(c) In lower motor neurone lesions of the facial nerve there may (depending on the site of the lesion) also be loss of taste and hyperacusis. Occasionally, as for example in the case of an intracranial lesion, there may be lesions of adjacent cranial nerves — particularly of cranial nerves V, VI and VIII. In upper motor neurone lesions of the facial nerve there may be pyramidal lesions, e.g. hemiplegia, dysarthria, etc.

(d) With systemic corticosteroids e.g. 40 mg prednisone daily, reducing over one week.

A 3.8   (a) Blue sclerae in osteogenesis imperfecta; the pigmented choroid shows through a thin sclera. There are other causes of blue sclerae including normal infants, Ehler's–Danlos syndrome, pseudoxanthoma elasticum, etc.

(b) Dentinogenesis imperfecta (see A2.7).

(c) (i) Progressive deafness (otosclerosis).
  (ii) The complications from recurrent multiple fractures — such as chest deformities.
  (iii) Mitral valve prolapse or aortic incompetence in some cases.
  (iv) Weakness of tendons and ligaments.

Osteogenesis imperfecta is a rare disorder, often inherited in autosomal dominant manner and characterized by fragile bones (Fragilitas ossium). Minimal trauma may cause fractures and deformities may result. Several subtypes have been described which vary in inheritance and severity (Table A3.8).

Table A3.8 Sub-types of Osteogenesis Imperfecta

Sub-type	Inheritance	Blue sclerae	Bone disease	Stature	Dentinogenesis imperfecta	Other comments
I	Autosomal dominant	+	Mild	Fairly normal	In a few	80 per cent are of this type. Also may have hypermobile joints and thin aortic valves.
II	Autosomal recessive	+	Severe	Lethal in neonate	Lethal in neonate	Lethal in neonate.
III	Autosomal recessive or sporadic	−	Severe	Reduced	In a few	. Progressive deformity.
IV	Autosomal dominant	−	Severe	Reduced	Common	Severe deformity.
V	Variable	−	Mild	Normal	Rare	Features of Ehlers – Danlos syndrome.

A 3.9 (a) Denture-induced stomatitis (denture sore mouth; chronic atrophic candidosis).

    (b) (i) The dentures should be checked for their adequacy.

       (ii) Dentures should be left out of the mouth at night, cleaned and stored in 1 per cent hypochlorite (Milton; Dentural).

       (iii) An antifungal agent applied to the denture fitting surface (e.g. miconazole oral gel) is helpful, or the patient can use amphotericin (Fungilin) lozenges 10 mg or nystatin tablets 500 000 units dissolved in the mouth 4 times daily. Miconazole cream is useful to treat any associated angular cheilitis.

    (c) Angular cheilitis (see A1.3).

Erythema confined to the denture-bearing area is almost invariably caused by chronic candidosis related to colonization with *Candida albicans*. Denture allergy is almost unknown. Denture stomatitis is usually asymptomatic and of little consequence unless associated with angular cheilitis. Papillary hyperplasia is an uncommon complication.

Angular cheilitis is almost invariably bilateral and characterized by soreness and erythema (sometimes with fissuring or ulceration) of the skin at the angles of the mouth. Most patients with angular cheilitis wear full dentures and have candidosis beneath the upper denture. There may also be inadequacies of the dentures.

Iron deficiency, riboflavin deficiency and other deficiency states are rare causes of angular cheilitis (see also A1.3).

A 3.10 (a) Inflamed operculum over $\overline{8|}$. Pyogenic granuloma adjacent to $\overline{7|}$.

(b) This is an example of the migratory abscess of the buccal sulcus in a case of acute pericoronitis tracking to emerge, usually, buccal to the first molar. In this case the lower first molar is absent and the second molar has drifted forward. Rarely, of course, there may be concurrent infection affecting more than one site with more than one cause. The appearance shown may therefore represent a lateral periodontal abscess occurring concurrently with an episode of acute pericoronitis affecting different teeth.

(c) Treatment of the acute pericoronitis. Primary treatment may involve the extraction of an opposing upper third molar which traumatizes the operculum and irrigation of the operculum with an astringent such as trichloracetic acid suitably buffered and the prescription of a course of antibiotics such as metronidazole or penicillin. Abscess drainage may occasionally be indicated in acute pericoronitis. Hot salt-water baths and analgesics are also indicated. Definitive treatment is very likely to comprise extraction of the lower third molar when the acute infection has subsided.

A 3.11 (a) A keloid scar.

(b) Collagen and fibroblasts. There is some evidence to suggest that some collagen types are present more frequently than others and that a tendency to keloid is associated with specific HLA tissue types. It certainly is more common in negroids, pregnant patients, and those with tuberculosis.

(c) 1. Surgical excision and skin grafting.
2. Surgical excision followed by an iridium implant into the resulting sutured wound.

3. Intra-lesional steroid injections. A large keloid scar such as this is unlikely to resolve completely by this means.
4. Surgical excision followed by cryosurgery to the healing wound approximately two weeks following surgery.

A 3.12 (a) (i) Cranio-maxillary fixation. This has been applied here by means of supra-orbital pins and external fixation. Cranio-maxillary fixation may also be applied internally by means of suspension wires. These methods have the advantage that the mouth is open for suction and airway control in the first few hours after operation. Intermaxillary fixation to restore the occlusion is nearly always necessary in the longer term.
(ii) Levant frame.

(b) Lead plates.

(c) 1. Nasal plaster.
2. Nasal packing.
3. Direct wiring.

(d) The ethmoid bone.

A 3.13 (a) Speckled leucoplakia.

(b) Up to 20 per cent show malignant change in 20 years: this leucoplakia has a worse prognosis than the more common homogeneous leucoplakia.

This lesion is speckled i.e. a mixture of red lesions (erythroplasia) with white lesions (leucoplakia). The red component is caused by epithelial atrophy and often shows dysplastic changes.

In any event, studies have shown that there is about a 10 per cent incidence of clinically unsuspected early carcinoma in leucoplakias and therefore a biopsy (in this instance of a red area) is indicated. Some of these lesions are associated with a heavy colonization by candida species.

A 3.14 (a) Paget's disease of bone (osteitis deformans).

(b) (i) Swelling of the affected jaw.
(ii) Hypercementosis (and subsequent difficulty with extractions).
(iii) Tendency to post-extraction haemorrhage and infection.

   (c) Serum alkaline phosphatase levels (raised). Calcium and phosphate levels (usually normal).

   (d) Calcitonin or diphosphonates.

Paget's disease is a common disorder, particularly in the elderly, and may have a viral aetiology. It is typified by enlargement of the skull, kyphosis, and bowed legs with a liability to pathological fractures and sarcoma. The skull thickens and may produce headache, facial pain, and disturbances of vision and hearing. About 15 per cent of patients have jaw involvement and a bony swelling (shown), pain and difficulty in wearing dentures.

   The cotton wool appearance on skull radiography is very characteristic of Paget's disease (see also A1.2).

A 3.15 (a) A pregnancy epulis (pyogenic granuloma).

   (b) A thorough scale and polish in this area may lead to a significant reduction in the volume of these lesions. Postpartum these lesions virtually always shrink away to nothing and no further treatment is required. However, they may assume a large size, as has occurred in this case, and may require surgical excision. This should be performed under local anaesthesia and a thorough scale and polish should be performed at the same time. The importance of thorough oral hygiene should be impressed on the patient as recurrence is a likely event in the presence of plaque and calculus deposits.

   (c) This is a common site for this lesion. In this area of the mouth the lower teeth frequently occlude on the palatal mucosa giving rise to trauma which adds to the reaction of the oedematous vascular mucosa to plaque and calculus.

PAPER 4

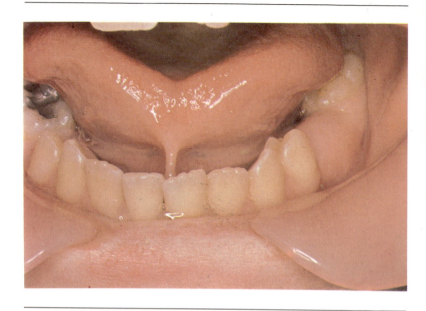

Q 4.1   (a) What is this condition?

(b) What problems may the patient have?

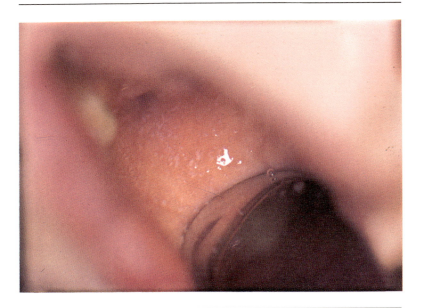

Q 4.2 This is the buccal mucosa in a child with a fever, a runny nose, and sore throat.

(a) What is the diagnosis?

(b) What is the most common serious complication of this condition?

(c) What is the cause?

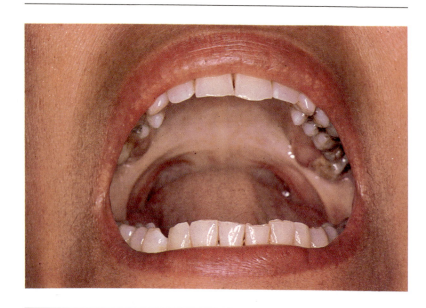

Q 4.3 This lady had trismus. Examination also revealed an immobile soft palate.

(a) What is the differential diagnosis?

(b) What is the prognosis?

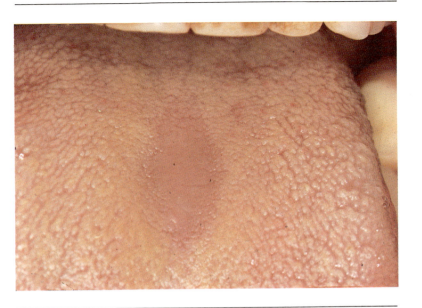

Q 4.4 (a) What is the probable diagnosis of this lesion on the dorsum of the tongue?

(b) What may be the aetiology?

(c) What are the histopathological features?

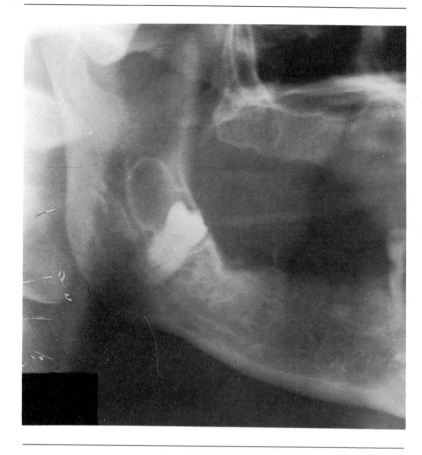

Q 4.5 (a) From the radiographic features seen here, which cyst type is most likely?

(b) How might aspiration of the cyst contents aid diagnosis?

(c) Name two radiographic features seen here which may indicate proximity of the inferior alveolar neurovascular bundle to 8̄| roots.

(d) Name two other radiographic features not seen here which might indicate close proximity of the neurovascular bundle to the wisdom tooth roots.

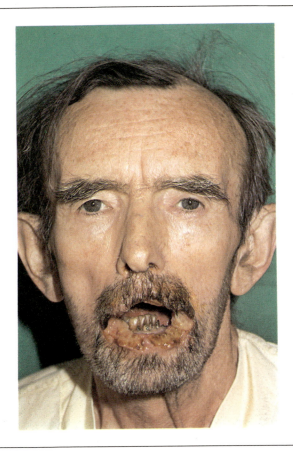

Q 4.6   (a) What disease process is represented here?

(b) What organism may be cultured from this lesion?

(c) Name five predisposing conditions.

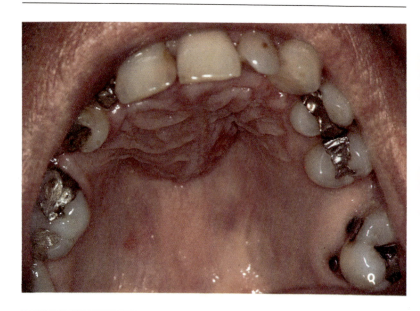

Q 4.7 This patient complained of severe throbbing pain and swelling in the anterior part of the maxilla.

(a) What is the likely diagnosis?

(b) Which teeth are likely to be involved?

(c) What is the treatment?

(d) What organisms are usually responsible for this condition?

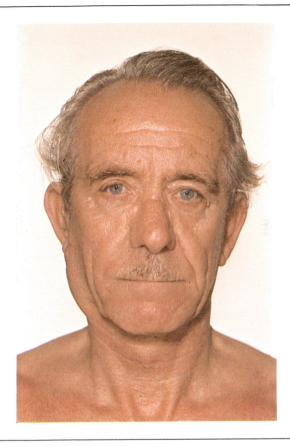

Q 4.8 (a) Which clinical sign most clearly indicates the origin of this swelling?

(b) The cause of this swelling was a malignant neoplasm. Which other signs may be demonstrated in such a patient?

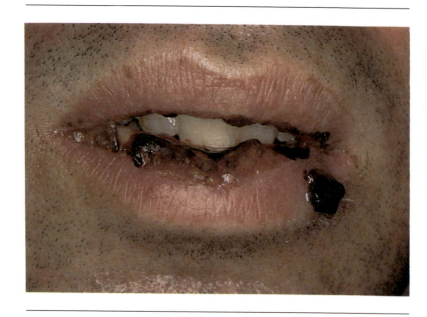

Q 4.9 (a) This is a characteristic presentation of which disease?

(b) What other tissues may be involved?

(c) What is known of the aetiology?

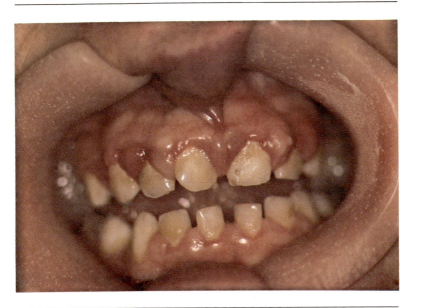

Q 4.10 (a) What is a likely exogenous cause of this problem?

(b) What other oral complications may be seen?

(c) What drugs should be avoided in patients with this condition?

(d) What drugs may cause similar complications?

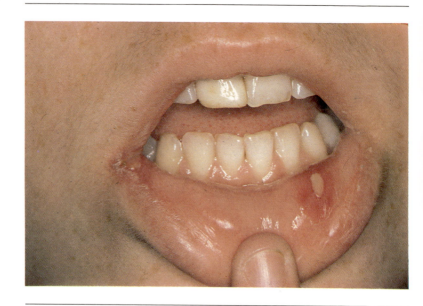

Q 4.11 (a) What is the probable diagnosis in this patient who suffered from frequent recurrent mouth ulcers?

    (b) What conditions should be excluded?

    (c) What useful local treatments are available?

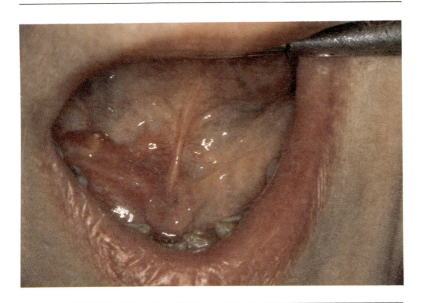

Q 4.12 This patient complained of pain in the floor of the mouth on the
right side, and submandibular swelling.

(a) How would you examine this region of the mouth?

(b) What investigations would you perform?

(c) What is the probable diagnosis?

(d) What is the treatment?

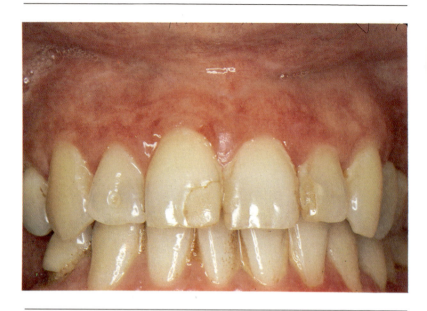

Q 4.13 This patient was referred by her dentist with a diagnosis of gingivitis.

(a) What are the possible diagnoses?

(b) How would you confirm the diagnosis?

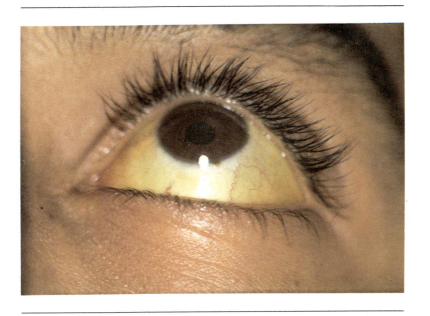

Q 4.14 (a) What is shown here?

(b) What are the main groups of causes?

(c) How may dental management be complicated?

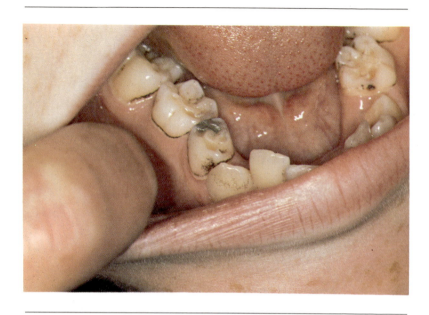

Q 4.15 (a) What is the probable cause of this tooth discoloration?

(b) What is the significance of it, if any?

A 4.1   (a) Ankyloglossia (tongue tie).

(b) Speech is *NOT* usually impaired. The patient may find difficulty in cleaning food from his labial vestibule and may consequently develop caries and/or periodontal disease.

Partial ankyloglossia appears to have a genetic basis and has a prevalence of 1 in 400 to 1 in 3000 births in various studies. Partial ankyloglossia is usually an isolated anomaly. Rarely there are associated syndromes such as orofaciodigital or cleft-lip/cleft palate/lip-pit syndrome.

NB $\overline{5|5}$ are unerupted

A 4.2   (a) Measles (these are Koplik's spots).

(b) Pneumonia. In Third World countries this causes significant morbidity and mortality (see also A4.6).

(c) Measles virus.

Koplik's spots appear on the buccal mucosa on the 2nd or 3rd day of measles, preceding the skin lesions by 1 or 2 days. Koplik's spots are usually seen in the mucosa close to the mandibular first molars. Caused by superficial necrosis, the spots resolve within one week.

Spots in the buccal mucosa in adults caused by ectopic sebaceous glands (Fordyce spots) should not be confused since they are yellow rather than white (see A1.11) and otherwise the patient is well.

A 4.3   (a) (i) Submucous fibrosis (she is Asian).
             (ii) Scleroderma.

(b) Submucous fibrosis is restricted to the oral tissues: it may have a premalignant potential.

This is submucous fibrosis (also known as oral submucous fibrosis: OSMF).

OSMF is a rare condition seen mainly in SE Asians and is somewhat more prevalent in females than males. The onset is insidious with a burning sensation followed by increasing stiffness of lips, tongue and palate, and concomitant trismus. The mucosa appears blanched and, in some areas, pigmented, over bands of tough fibrous tissue.

The condition appears to be dietary (?chillies) in origin but there may be a genetic predisposition.

A 4.4   (a) Median rhomboid glossitis.

(b) May be congenital (persistence of the tuberculum impar) or may be associated with candidal infection. Smoking may predispose to the candidosis.

(c) There is:
(i) absence of filiform papillae.
(ii) epithelial hyperplasia and acanthosis.
(iii) chronic inflammatory infiltrate in the lamina propria.
The epithelial hyperplasia may be pseudoepitheliomatous. This has, in the past, led to the misdiagnosis of this lesion as carcinoma.

The slightly rhomboidal, red, depapillated area is in the midline, just anterior to the circumvallate papilla — the characteristic site for median rhomboid glossitis. This is an uncommon lesion, with a predilection for males, and with a good prognosis.

A 4.5 (a) Follicular or lateral dentigerous cyst. The defunct follicle around the crown of any unerupted tooth (but especially in this region) may commence bone-resorbing prostaglandin production leading to cyst formation.

(b) The aspirate can be subjected to electrophoresis and proteins identified. In this case the most important distinction to be made is between a follicular cyst and a keratocyst. Keratocysts often recur after cyst enucleation, unless precautions are taken (for example spraying of resulting bony cavities with liquid nitrogen to kill residual cells). Therefore, it is useful to know the precise diagnosis prior to operation. In keratocysts, protein concentration will be less than 4 g/100 ml and in follicular cysts greater than 5 g/100 ml cyst fluid.

(c) A change in direction of the inferior dental canal and superimposition of the roots on the canal outline.

If there is proximity of roots to the canal there may be damage to its contents during tooth extraction with consequent labial anaesthesia or paraesthesia.

(d) Narrowing of the inferior dental bundle may indicate proximity. Loss of the radio-opaque outline of the inferior dental bundle is a radiographic sign often referred to in the literature, but is not reliable. Orthopantomograms are notorious in their lack of detail in this respect and, even using other radiographic views (for example, the lateral oblique film), these two radio-opaque lines may be lost due to superimposition of the third molar roots and the variable course of the bundle in relation to the cortices and medulla of the mandible.

A 4.6   (a) Cancrum oris (Noma).

Carcinoma must be excluded.

   (b) Commensal organisms from mouth and skin. It is assumed that
       cancrum oris is an extension of acute ulcerative gingivitis in
       debilitated patients but this has yet to be conclusively demons-
       trated.

   (c) Common predisposing factors in the tropics are measles,
       mumps, malnutrition, and malaria. Any disease which severely
       compromises the immune system may be the precursor to
       cancrum oris, and this case illustrates cancrum oris affecting a
       patient with acute myelofibrosis. Cancrum oris may also (rare-
       ly) affect leukaemics.
          In the second case, illustrated here (Fig. A4.6), the disease
       process has terminated, leaving severe scarring and contrac-
       ture. Circumoral muscles have been destroyed, rendering the
       area difficult to reconstruct with soft-tissue flaps.

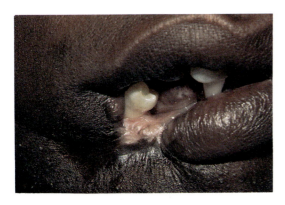

Fig. A4.6

A 4.7   (a) Dental abscess (acute periapical abscess).

   (b) This dento-alveolar abscess almost certainly arises from $\underline{2|}$.
       Upper lateral incisor roots are usually (but not always) inclined
       palatally so that pus, taking the path of least resistance, is most
       likely to burst through the palatal bone. Abscesses related to
       other upper anterior teeth usually point on the buccal side of
       the alveolus.

   (c) Incision and drainage. Local analgesia may be achieved using
       ethyl chloride spray or other topical analgesic. It is sometimes

possible to combine incision and drainage with removal of the lateral incisor by infiltrating local anaesthetic solution buccally, adjacent to the upper lateral incisor. However, extraction of the incisor root is normally postponed until local infection is under control. General anaesthesia is rarely justified for such a procedure, except in a child. Drainage may be achieved by making an incision antero-posteriorly approximately 1 cm in length over the most dependent part of the swelling. In this site there is unlikely to be more than one locule of pus so that Hilton's technique need not be employed. Culture and sensitivity testing of the resulting pus very rarely provides information which is of practical use. Antibiotics are indicated only if symptoms do not resolve after free drainage has been achieved, and the cause of the abscess eliminated.

(d) Most studies indicate that about half of these abscesses are caused by a specific micro-organism, commonly *viridans streptococci* which are common oral commensals. *Staphylococcus aureus* appears to be the next most commonly incriminated. Non-haemolytic streptococci and anaerobic streptococci may also be involved. Mixed infections have also been reported involving streptococcus, staphylococcus, fusobacterium, and other organisms.

Dental caries or trauma to teeth (including dental procedures) are the common causes of pulp necrosis which is a prelude to the formation of an abscess at the apex of the tooth. This produces severe persistent throbbing pain that is worse on biting or touching the tooth. Intraoral and facial swelling are not uncommon.

A 4.8 (a) Eversion of the ear lobe on the right side. This is virtually pathognomonic of parotid gland pathology. Unusually, this lesion turned out to be a secondary deposit from carcinoma of the bronchus, involving the parotid gland.

(b) Other signs of malignant parotid pathology include pain, duct obstruction, trismus, paralysis of the muscles of facial expression secondary to facial nerve involvement, and signs of infiltration of glossopharyngeal, vagus, accessory, and hypoglossal nerves, if deep aspects are involved. Disturbances in sensation in areas innervated by the great auricular and auriculo-temporal nerves may also be features.

Mumps is the most common cause of swelling, particularly in children, and this is more commonly bilateral than unilateral. Parotid swelling is also seen in ascending bacterial sialadenitis, salivary duct obstruction, Sjogren's syndrome, neoplasms, sarcoidosis, and with some drugs.

Neoplasms are not uncommon and are predominantly pleomorphic salivary adenoma, usually a benign neoplasm.

A 4.9   (a) Erythema multiforme.

      (b) Other mucosa and skin (also, rarely, the joints.)

      (c) An aetiological agent is frequently not identified. Some cases appear to be an allergic type of reaction to micro-organisms (herpes simplex; mycoplasma) or drugs (barbiturates; sulphonamides, etc.). Circulating immune complexes have been found in many patients with erythema multiforme (see also A2.9).

Blood-stained crusting of the lips with severe oral ulceration, in a young male, is not uncommonly caused by erythema multiforme. The lesions of the other vesiculobullous disorders (e.g. pemphigus), usually do not bleed and, in those that may bleed (e.g. mucous membrane pemphigoid), the lesions in general are more circumscribed and affect areas more posteriorly in the mouth.

Ocular, genital, nasal, and urethral mucosa may be involved and if this is the case and the patient has a fever, the condition is known as Steven–Johnson syndrome.

A 4.10   (a) Phenytoin (Epanutin: Dilantin).

      (b) (i) Trauma to hard or soft tissues during epileptic convulsions.
          (ii) Phenytoin may, rarely, cause folate deficiency (predisposing to oral ulceration).

      (c) Epileptogenic drugs such as methohexitone, tricyclics and phenothiazines (e.g. chlorpromazine).

      (d) Cyclosporine and nifedipine may also produce gingival hyperplasia.

Gingival hyperplasia may be present to a minor degree in patients with chronic marginal gingivitis. Generalized hyperplasia may be drug-induced (e.g. phenytoin) or may be idiopathic or inherited. Hereditary forms may be autosomal dominant and may be associated with hypertrichosis. Rare conditions such as the mucopolysaccharidoses and mucolipidoses, especially I cell disease, may cause gingival hyperplasia.

Phenytoin hyperplasia is more likely to occur where oral hygiene is poor and begins with hyperplasia of the gingival papillae (shown). The gingivae may occasionally become so hyperplastic that the teeth become buried.

A 4.11 (a) Minor aphthous ulcers.

(b) (i) Haematological deficiencies.
(ii) Malabsorption states.
(iii) Behcet's disease.

(c) (i) Chlorhexidine 0.2 per cent aqueous mouthwash.
(ii) Topical corticosteroids:
Adcortyl in orabase (triamcinolone acetonide).
Corlan (hydrocortisone hemisuccinate 2.5 mg. pellets, one used 4 times daily), and many others.

These are the common type of ulcers. They are recurrent ulcers that begin in childhood or adolescence. Patients usually have 1 to 6 ulcers at any episode. The ulcers affect particularly the labial and buccal mucosa and the vestibule but may also affect the floor of the mouth/ventrum of tongue. Minor aphthous ulcers rarely affect the palate or dorsum of tongue. The ulcers heal in about 5–10 days. Minor aphthous ulcers are, as shown here, round or ovoid circumscribed ulcers with a yellow base and an erythematous halo. They are 2–4 mm in diameter. Two ulcers are shown here.

A 4.12 (a) Using bi-manual palpation. The tissues in the floor of the mouth are arranged loosely, so that pressure to the region results in displacement of lumps and stones, giving little information. This can be prevented by the simple expedient of pressure on the submandibular skin from the other hand.

(b) Lower occlusal radiographs to demonstrate the stone seen here under the mucosa in the $\overline{6|}$ region. Radiography is not superfluous in these obvious cases because further stones may be present anteriorly or posteriorly. (Not all are radio-opaque).

(c) Submandibular sialolithiasis (calculus). This is commonly due to stasis in the gland after upper respiratory tract infections or other pyrexic episodes. Stasis may also follow sialadenitis, sometimes after irradiation to the head and neck. Sialolithiasis appears to be unrelated to a defined disorder of calcium metabolism or to the occurrence of calculi elsewhere in the body.

(d) These stones may be removed from an intraoral approach under local anaesthesia if they present in this site. Stones presenting more posteriorly may necessitate excision of the submandibular gland. Local anaesthetic is infiltrated around the stone and also further posteriorly. A stay suture is then looped around the duct posteriorly to prevent displacement back into the gland when surgical removal is attempted. An incision over the stone and parallel to the submandibular duct is then made down to the stone, which can then be removed. Sutures are not usually necessary to repair the resulting defect.

A 4.13 (a) Desquamative gingivitis. This is usually caused by
    (i) lichen planus
    (ii) pemphigoid or
    (iii) pemphigus
    but *NOT* by the menopause (in contrast to traditional views).

  (b) (i) Examination for lesions elsewhere on mucosa or skin.
    (ii) Biopsy.
    (iii) Immunological investigations.

The term 'gingivitis' usually refers to marginal gingivitis i.e. erythema and swelling of the gingival margins and papillae, related to the accumulation on the teeth of dental bacterial plaque, because of poor hygiene. In this patient the erythema affects the whole gingiva, extending into the vestibule. The erythema is patchy and caused by epithelial loss rather than inflammation *per se* i.e. it is desquamative.

NB $\underline{21|12}$ have tooth-coloured restoratious; $\dfrac{2|}{4|}$ are carious.

A 4.14 (a) Jaundice (yellow or icteric sclerae).

  (b) (i) Biliary obstruction (e.g. gallstones; cancer of pancreas).
    (ii) Liver disease (e.g. hepatitis).
    (iii) Haemolysis (e.g. sickle cell anaemia).

  (c) Depending on the cause, there may be:
    (i) Bleeding tendency.
    (ii) Problems with drug handling (especially with general anaesthesia).
    (iii) Danger of cross infection e.g. with hepatitis viruses.

A 4.15 (a) Black stain.

  (b) A lower caries incidence is found.

Black stain is of uncertain aetiology in most cases.

Drugs such as iron or foods such as liquorice or betel may cause black stain but most children with black stain have no known predisposing cause.

In some parts of the world, teeth are deliberately stained with herbs, lacquers, etc. Usually the stain is used for cosmetic reasons alone, occasionally for more deliberate purposes (e.g. Japanese prostitutes!).

PAPER 5

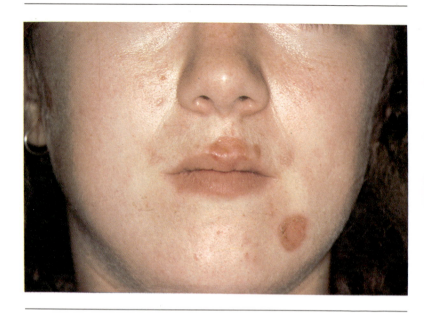

Q 5.1 (a) What is the diagnosis?

(b) Outline the natural history of this disorder.

(c) What is the treatment?

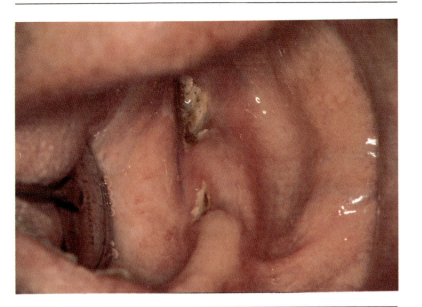

Q 5.2   This 78 year old man had a squamous cell carcinoma affecting the tongue, which was treated by radiotherapy ten years prior to this photograph. He attended for adjustment to his full dentures and had noticed only very mild discomfort affecting the alveolus in the region shown.

(a) What is the likely cause of the exposed bone shown here?

(b) What are the radiographic features which may be seen in this condition?

(c) Which tissues does this condition affect?

(d) In the absence of evidence of widespread disease, how may this particular patient's condition be managed?

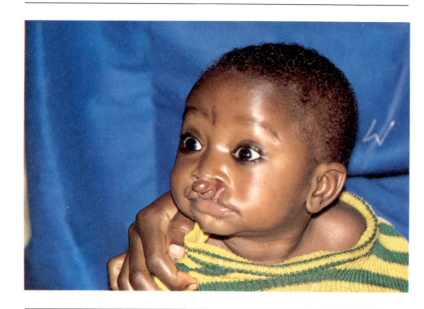

Q 5.3 This baby was brought to hospital with a bilateral cleft lip.

(a) Is a cleft lip on its own more likely to occur in a girl or a boy?

(b) Is the incidence of associated congenital malformation greatest in a child with a cleft lip or a cleft palate.

(c) What abnormalities in maxillary growth may be expected in a patient with a complete cleft palate?

(d) List the dental abnormalities which can be expected to accompany an alveolar cleft.

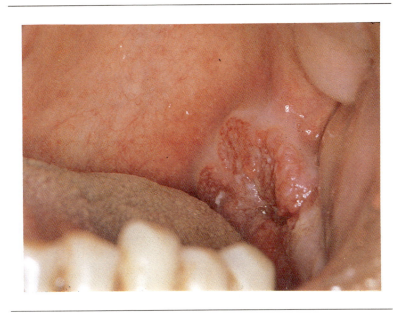

Q 5.4   (a) What is the probable diagnosis?

(b) How would you investigate this patient?

(c) What drug treatment is available?

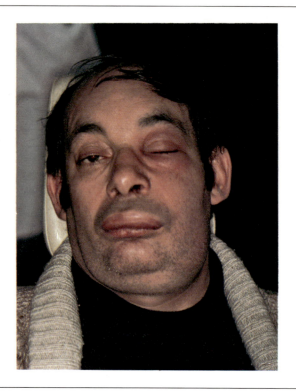

Q 5.5 This 42 year old man presented with a painful swelling of the upper left face and circumorbital oedema.

(a) What is the most likely oral cause?

(b) By which route may organisms from a maxillary infection enter the cavernous sinus?

(c) What are the principal signs associated with cavernous sinus thrombosis?

(d) How may cavernous sinus thrombosis be treated?

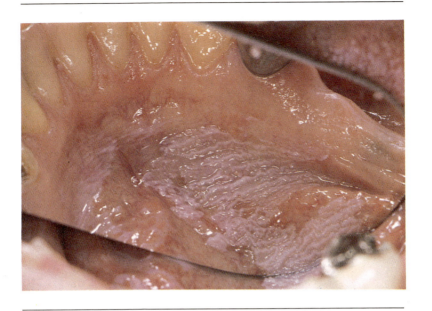

Q 5.6   (a) What is this lesion?

(b) What is the prognosis?

(c) How would you manage the patient?

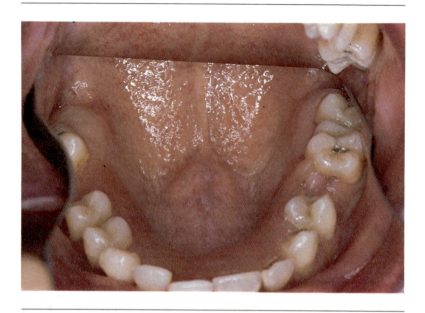

Q 5.7   This patient noticed a hard lump in the palate. What is the probable diagnosis?

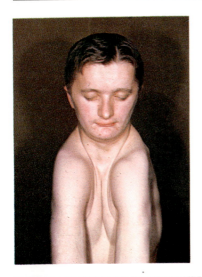

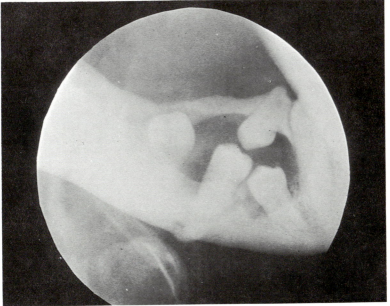

Q 5.8   (a) What is the diagnosis?

(b) What oral lesions may occur?

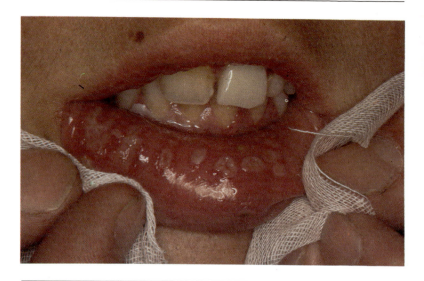

Q 5.9 This chemistry student complained of fever, malaise, sore throat, 'glands' in the neck, sore gums, and mouth ulcers.

(a) What is the probable diagnosis?

(b) What may be the outcome if the patient has eczema?

(c) How would you manage this patient?

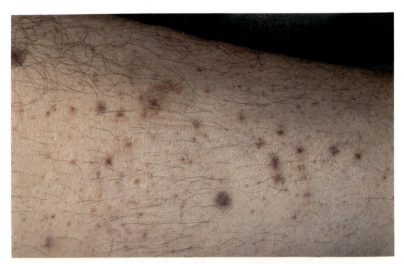

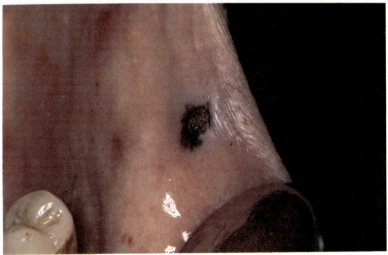

Q 5.10 This patient complained of gingival bleeding and was noted to have these lesions. The lesions did not blanch on pressure.

(a) What is the problem here?

(b) What are possible causes?

(c) How would you investigate the patient's condition?

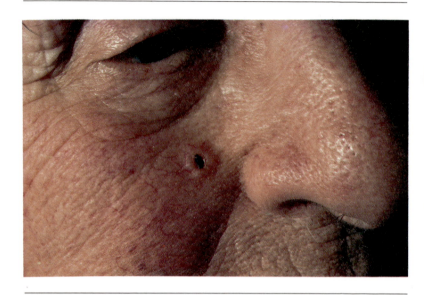

Q 5.11 (a) What is the probable diagnosis?

    (b) Is this a common site for this particular lesion?

    (c) What is the treatment?

    (d) What is the differential diagnosis?

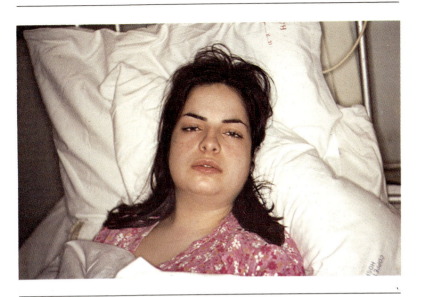

Q 5.12 This lady had trismus fever and painful parotid swellings.

(a) What is the probable cause?

(b) What other glands apart from salivary glands may be affected?

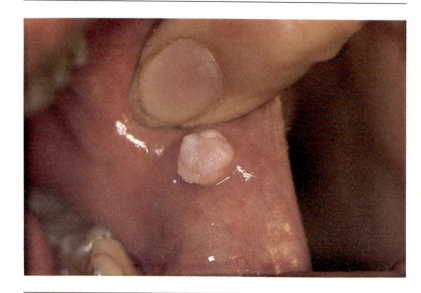

Q 5.13 (a) What is the probable diagnosis of this virally induced lesion?

(b) How would you manage this patient?

(c) What viruses are implicated and what other oral lesions might they induce?

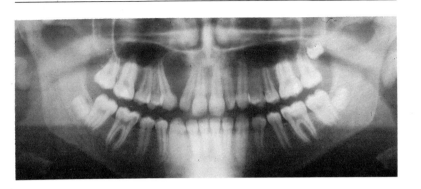

Q 5.14 This radiograph is from a 14 year old girl.

    (a) What abnormality is shown here?

    (b) All standing teeth were vital. Give a differential diagnosis.

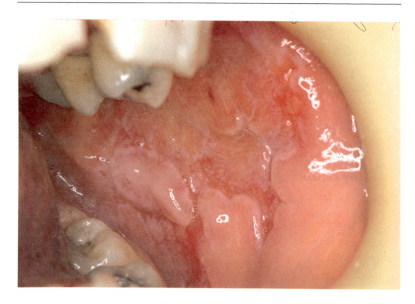

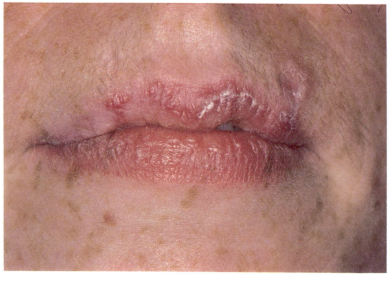

Q 5.15 These lesions are in the same patient.

(a) What is the probable diagnosis?

(b) What are the histopathological features?

A 5.1   (a) Impetigo contagiosa.

(b) This bacterial infection usually starts with bulla formation under the stratum corneum. These bullae soon discharge onto the skin surface where yellowish crusting occurs due to drying out of the bulla contents.

(c) Crusts should be removed with warm water and the skin allowed to dry. Once or twice daily applications of Neomycin or Fucidin cream should then be instituted. Topical antibiotics are usually sufficient in mild cases but more severe infection may warrant systemic antimicrobial therapy with flucloxacillin.

Impetigo is a highly contagious bacterial infection and lesions spread easily to other areas of the body. Impetigo may also complicate facial skin lesions such as herpes labialis and chickenpox. The organisms responsible include the staphylococcus aureus or beta haemolytic streptococcus. Staphylococcus phage types nos. 71, 80, and 81 are the most likely to be involved.

A 5.2   (a) Osteoradionecrosis.

(b) Osteoradionecrosis usually gives rise to patchy radiopacity in the area affected (see Fig. A5.2). This may occur in the absence of infection although further radiographic changes are usually the result of osteomyelitis rather than simply osteoradionecrosis. Evidence of periosteal new bone formation is less likely in the osteomyelitis which follows irradiation, due to endarteritis affecting this area.

(c) Radiation therapy affects all tissues to a greater or lesser extent and endarteritis obliterans commonly affects mucoperiosteum as well as bone. As far as soft tissue is concerned, irradiation produces obliteration of the small vascular channels rendering some of the tissue hypoxic. The tissue responds by a decrease in volume giving rise to, for example, a markedly thinner mucoperiosteal layer. Bone is unable to respond in such a fashion due to its calcified component and is therefore more susceptible to infection and further necrosis.

(d) The status of the surrounding bone may be investigated by means of plain radiographic examination and scintigraphy.
      In the absence of symptoms, it is often best not to carry out any active treatment. Surgical intervention should be carried out with extreme caution due to the possible widespread nature of the radionecrosis. 'Let sleeping dogs lie' is an appropriate

maxim here. If surgical débridement is undertaken then prophylactic antibiotics should be given orally or intramuscularly. Extensive soft tissue repair is not indicated, due to local endarteritis obliterans, and mucosa should be left to reform by secondary intention after sequestrectomy.

Hyperbaric oxygen may have a place in the management of this condition, especially if intractable low grade osteomyelitis ensues. Occasionally, extensive mandibular resections are the only option in widespread infection. Reconstruction after such procedures should involve the grafting of vital bone and soft tissues preferably using vascularized tissue and microvascular techniques.

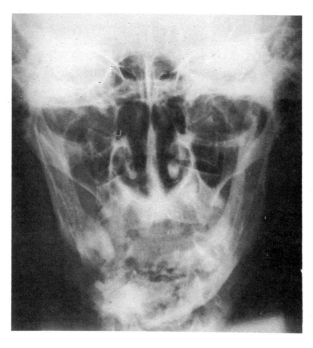

Fig. A5.2

A 5.3   (a) Cleft lips are more common in boys.

    (b) Associated congenital defects such as spina bifida and hypospadias are more common in patients with cleft palates.

    (c) Apart from local dental abnormalities associated with alveolar clefts, maxillary hypoplasia is rarely seen except in so far as the cleft widens during growth. Secondary surgical correction of maxillary hypoplasia is often necessary however, because growth is inhibited due to the scarring which follows cleft repair as a baby.

(d) (i) Abnormalities in tooth number. These include absence of the ipsilateral deciduous and permanent lateral incisors and supernumerary lateral incisors. In one reported series, nearly 30 per cent of patients were without at least one tooth. Cases of hypodontia and anodontia have been reported.

(ii) Abnormalities of tooth form. Tuberculate lateral incisors and supernumerary incisors have been reported. Variations in size have also been encountered.

(iii) Abnormalities of tooth structure. Enamel hypoplasia, particularly affecting lateral incisors, frequently follows surgical repair of the alveolus in cleft cases. It is unclear whether hypoplasia is secondary simply to the alveolar cleft, or to the surgery used to repair the defect.

A 5.4 (a) This is a squamous cell carcinoma arising from the anterior pillar of the fauces.

(b) (i) A thorough physical examination with special emphasis on cervical lymphadenopathy, evidence of bilateral spread and nerve involvement. An incisional biopsy should be performed under local anaesthesia to confirm quickly the nature of this lesion.

(ii) Radiographic examination should involve intraoral periapical views and postero-anterior, lateral oblique, and occipitomental views. Tomographic examination may be of secondary use in these patients.

(iii) Computerized axial tomography. This will provide further information on soft tissue spread and lymph node involvement.

(iv) Scintigraphic scanning. These techniques will identify areas of increased cellular activity and thus provide information on tumour site particularly with reference to lymph node involvement. The real benefit of these methods has, however, recently been called into question. Other positive evidence of spread should be sought prior to treatment planning.

(c) Intravenous agents such as bleomycin and methotrexate may be delivered to the tumour site either intravenously or by local arterial route. In this case, cytotoxic agents may be perfused into the required areas from a cannula inserted into the external carotid artery. Chemotherapy is *far* less effective than radiotherapy or surgery (see A6.5).

A 5.5   (a) A dentoalveolar abscess associated with ⌊3.

(b) Organisms may be carried from this region to the cavernous sinus through the angular veins of the orbit.

(c) Patients with cavernous sinus thrombosis are usually severely pyrexic and the nerves passing through the sinus and its walls are affected to a greater or lesser extent. These nerves are:
  (i) Abducens nerve: Lateral rectus function may be affected and palsy may be the presenting neurological symptom in these patients.
  (ii) Trochlear nerve: Superior oblique muscle function may be affected on its own.
  (iii) Oculomotor: Ophthalmoplegia, pupil dilatation, and ptosis may therefore be features.
  (iv) Maxillary nerve. Paraesthesia affecting any of the branches of this nerve may be a feature.
  Obstruction to venous return may give rise to pulsating exophthalmos and oedema of periorbital tissues. This is usually severely painful.

(d) Cavernous sinus thrombosis is managed with immediate intravenous antibiotics, modified on the culture and sensitivity of pus from the facial lesion, when this information becomes available.

Any infective lesions affecting the area inferior to the eye and superior to the upper lip may, conceivably, give rise to this serious condition.

Organisms may also be conveyed to the cavernous sinus via veins of the pterygoid plexus in infections of the infratemporal fossa.

A 5.6   (a) Sublingual keratosis.

(b) The malignant potential of this sublingual floor-of-mouth keratosis is greater than most other white patches and has been estimated to be as high as 50 per cent in *some* studies. Certainly the premalignant potential is far greater than that of white patches (leucoplakia; keratosis) in general, which is about 3–5 per cent.

(c) Biopsy of red areas particularly (this type of keratosis frequently is a speckled type of leucoplakia) and frequent regular checks
with photographic records and biopsy of any suspicious area.

This sublingual, or floor-of-mouth keratosis, has a predilection for females
and is most common in late middle age. The clinical appearance is of a white,
or white and red, lesion, usually in the anterior floor of mouth and ventrum
of tongue. The surface is often wrinkled, giving the 'ebbing tide' appearance
shown well in this illustration.

Increased uptake by dysplastic areas of vital dyes, such as toluidine blue,
has been described and application may therefore have some place in
establishing the best site for biopsy. Definitive management may include
surgical excision and split skin grafting, cryosurgery, or laser therapy.
Malignant transformation in isolated cases has been reported following both
surgery and cryosurgery and it therefore seems important that longterm
follow-up is arranged in the same way as would be the case if no treatment
had been instituted.

A 5.7   Torus palatinus.

Torus palatinus is a fairly common, benign, bony excrescence in the middle
of the vault of the hard palate that usually first appears after puberty. There
is a slight female predisposition and there appears to be a genetic back-
ground. The prevalence is high amongst mongoloid peoples.

Torus palatinus is of little or no consequence but occasionally interferes
with denture construction and may require removal. Tori may also occur on
the lingual aspect of the mandible in the premolar region (torus mandibu-
laris).

A 5.8   (a) Cleidocranial dysostosis.

(b) (i) Unerupted teeth in both dentitions.
(ii) Supernumerary teeth.
(iii) Dentigerous cysts (follicular cysts).
(iv) Gemination and dilaceration.
The roots of the teeth appear to lack cellular cementum, a fact
that presumably explains the retarded eruption.

Cleidocranial dysostosis is a rare condition, often autosomal dominant,
characterized by clavicular hypoplasia or aplasia, brachycephaly with a wide
transverse diameter of the cranium and pronounced frontal and parietal
bossing (shown), a groove over the metopic suture (shown) and dental
anomalies (see (b)). Many other bony anomalies, such as poor development
of paranasal sinuses, may be present.

A 5.9 (a) Acute herpetic stomatitis (secondary syphilis, other viral infections, and acute leukaemia should be excluded). The scattered oval and round discrete ulcers are fairly characteristic (if there is fever and gingivitis) of herpes simplex stomatitis. Herpetic infections are decreasing in frequency and are affecting an increasingly older age group. Oral lesions may be caused by Type 1 or Type 2 herpes simplex virus and there may be venereal transmission.

(b) There may be widespread skin lesions of herpes simplex infection (eczema herpeticum), when antiviral therapy is indicated.

(c) (i) Soft diet.
(ii) Analgesics or a topical local anaesthetic such as 2 per cent viscous lignocaine solution.
(iii) Antipyretic.
(iv) Chlorhexidine 0.2 per cent mouthwash, or perhaps a tetracycline mouthbath.
(v) Antivirals — in the immunosuppressed patient (Acyclovir).

NB $\lfloor 1$ is crowned.

A 5.10 (a) Purpura.

(b) Platelet defect or, usually, deficiency as for example in autoimmune thrombocytopenia or bone marrow disease. This patient had leukaemia.

(c) Full blood picture and platelet count.
Platelets in health are in excess of about $150 \times 10^9/l$. Platelet function tests may be indicated. A Hess test may be of some value.

Gingival bleeding is a very common problem — usually associated with gingivitis or periodontitis — inflammatory diseases related to the accumulation of dental bacterial plaque. However, if oral petechiae are found in a patient with ready bleeding from or into the gingiva, thrombocytopenia may be responsible. Occasional petechiae may be either traumatic in origin, or rarely, found in amyloid disease.

A 5.11 (a) This lesion is a basal cell carcinoma. This particular lesion demonstrates the typical heaped-up beaded edge and superficial telangiectatic vessels.

(b) This is a very common site for this lesion. These lesions often present on the skin of the middle third of the face and also on other areas often exposed to sunlight. They are common in caucasians in sunny climes such as parts of Australia.

(c) This lesion would be treated by surgical excision, or radiotherapy.

(d) Keratoacanthoma: squamous cell carcinoma.

A 5.12 (a) Mumps.

    (b) (i) Pancreas
       (ii) Ovaries (testes in males).

Mumps is the most common cause of salivary gland swelling. It is an acute viral sialadenitis that predominantly affects children (usually the parotid glands, bilaterally). Occasionally mumps is unilateral or may affect the submandibular glands in isolation or in addition to the parotitis.

The salivary gland swelling is smooth-surfaced, tender, and associated with trismus, malaise, and fever, but no pus can be expressed from the salivary ducts. Diagnosis is on clinical findings although serology may be useful in diagnosis. Treatment is symptomatic only.

Other inflammatory causes of salivary gland swelling include bacterial sialadenitis, Sjögren's syndrome, and sarcoidosis (the latter two may cause bilateral parotid swelling). Sialosis may cause painless salivary gland swelling.

A 5.13 (a) Squamous cell papilloma.

    (b) Excision biopsy.

    (c) Human papilloma viruses (HPV).

The palate is a more common site for squamous cell papilloma that characteristically is a cauliflower-like exophytic pedunculated lesion. Multiple papillomas (not associated with HPV) characterize the focal dermal hypoplasia syndrome (Goltz syndrome) in which there are also cutaneous atrophy and pigmentation, iris colobomas, and various osseous anomalies.

HPV are implicated in verrucae, condyloma acuminatum, and in focal epithelial hyperplasia (Heck's disease).

HPV may be implicated in some leucoplakias and have recently been implicated in oral carcinoma.

A 5.14 (a) There is a radiolucency between 32| which has a smooth, well defined outline.

(b) In the presence of non-vital teeth, the most likely diagnosis is a dental cyst associated most probably with 2|. When all the teeth are vital however, this diagnosis is most unlikely. The possibilities are:

(i) Globulo-maxillary cyst. The true globulo-maxillary cyst is rare, developmental in origin and arises from epithelial cell nests at the site of embryonic fusion of maxilla and premaxilla.

(ii) Lateral periodontal cyst. Lateral periodontal cysts arise from odontogenic cell rests of Malassez in the periodontal membrane.

(iii) Residual cyst arising from C|. Residual cysts occur after teeth are extracted in the presence of a dental cyst. In the vast majority of cases, the dental cyst is effectively marsupialized into the mouth at the time of the extraction and disappears. When extraction is not accompanied by marsupialization, then cyst growth is likely to continue.

(iv) Odontogenic keratocyst. Keratocysts very often develop daughter micro-cysts which may give rise to recurrence at any time after enucleation of the major, parent, lesion.

It was thought that this possibly represented a true globulo-maxillary cyst lined with pseudostratified ciliated (respiratory) epithelium. However, enucleation was performed under local anaesthesia and the cyst lining found to be exceedingly thin. Histological examination revealed that this was in fact an odontogenic keratocyst. No further treatment was instituted and four months later there was there was evidence of bony healing. Longterm follow up was arranged.

NB 8| is missing and 6|6 are carious.

A 5.15 (a) Discoid lupus erythematosus (DLE).

(b) The histopathological features of DLE include:
(i) parakeratosis or hyperkeratosis
(ii) hydropic degeneration of the basal layer of epithelium
(iii) a dense perivascular mononuclear cell infiltrate
(iv) collagen degeneration beneath the epithelium and perivascularly (stains with periodic acid–Schiff).

This is *not* lichen planus (LP) although the buccal lesions resemble LP. However, the buccal ulcer has a periphery of closely packed parallel white striae rather than the more reticular type of lesion of LP. Lesions on the lips which are raised with a central scale are typical of DLE. However, the oral lesions of LP and DLE can be difficult to differentiate and each can resemble keratosis (leucoplakia). The presence of skin lesions in LP or DLE may help in making the diagnosis. Some 25 per cent of patients with cutaneous DLE have oral lesions; most patients with oral DLE have skin lesions.

NB $\overline{67}$ are carious.

PAPER 6

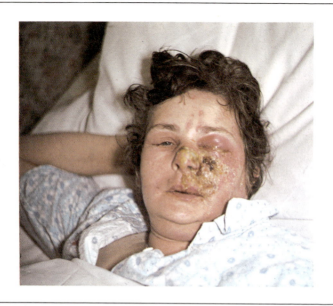

Q 6.1   (a) What is the diagnosis?

(b) What is the cause?

(c) What complications may occur?

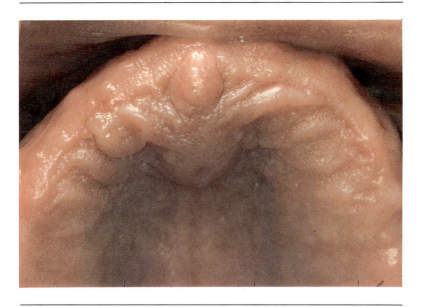

Q 6.2   What is the probable cause of this fluctuant swelling?

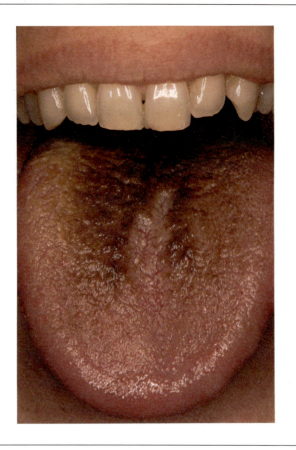

Q 6.3   (a) What is this condition?

      (b) What may be some causes?

      (c) How can it be treated?

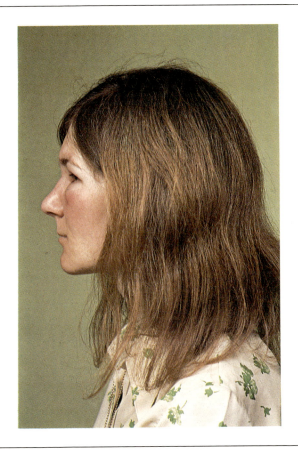

Q 6.4   This patient complained of facial swelling (as shown) after dental treatment on several occasions.

    (a) What conditions should be considered?

    (b) What investigations may be indicated?

    (c) What is the potential danger of such a reaction?

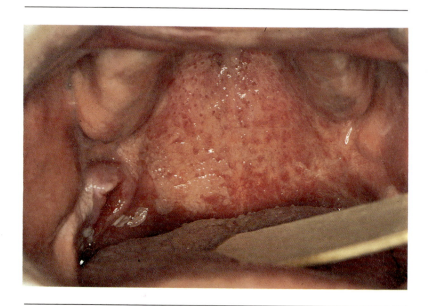

Q 6.5   This patient was a pipe smoker, referred by his dentist, who had noted a white lesion in the palate.

(a) What is the probable diagnosis?

(b) How would you manage this patient?

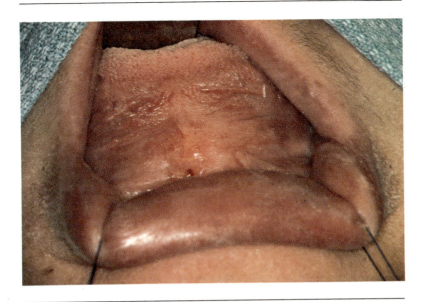

Q 6.6   This photograph shows the upwardly displaced tongue of a 58 year old patient who complained of mild hoarseness and dysphagia over the last year.

(a) How would you investigate this lesion?

(b) What is the differential diagnosis?

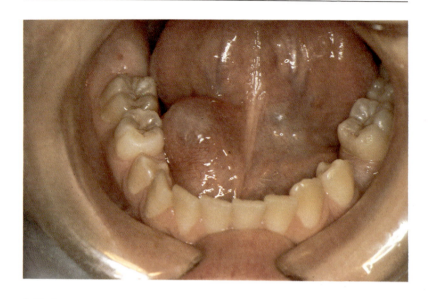

Q 6.7 (a) What is this lesion?

(b) Which structure usually limits the inferior extension of this lesion?

(c) What is the treatment?

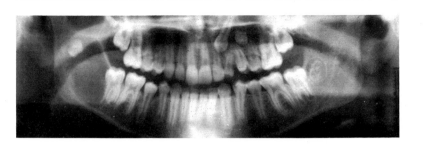

Q 6.8 (a) What radiographic abnormalities are seen here?

(b) Are further radiographs usually necessary for the localization of ⌊3?

(c) Comment on the positions of the third molar teeth.

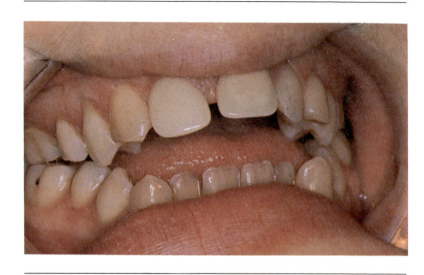

Q 6.9 (a) Name two possible causes of this malocclusion.

(b) Is this appearance indicative of an underlying pathologic process?

(c) What condition is illustrated here?

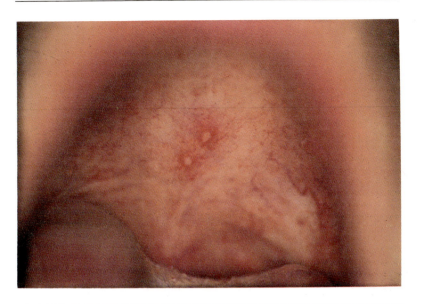

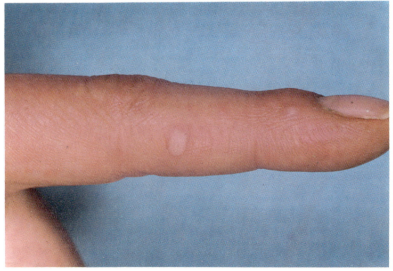

Q 6.10 (a) What is this condition?

(b) What is the cause?

(c) Which group of patients does it normally affect?

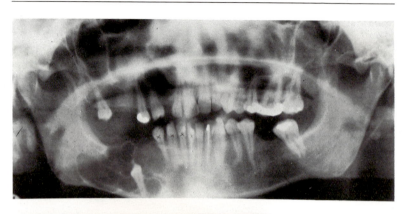

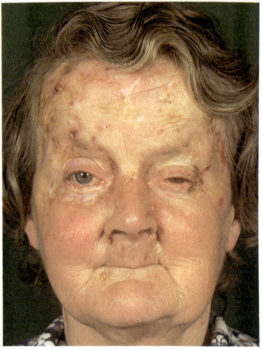

Q 6.11 This patient had had several mandibular cysts removed. A panoramic radiograph of the jaws and a clinical slide are shown.

(a) What is the diagnosis?

(b) What other radiographs might be useful?

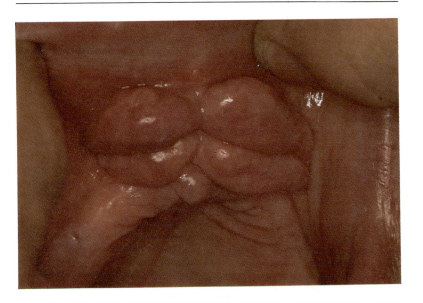

Q 6.12 (a) What is this condition?

(b) What is the treatment?

(c) What is the incidence of malignant change in this condition?

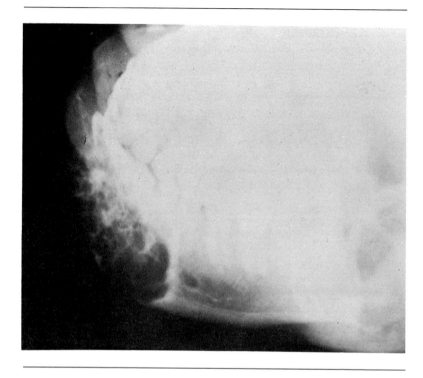

Q 6.13 This lateral oblique radiograph shows evidence of a lesion affecting the mandible.

(a) Give a differential diagnosis.

(b) How might aspiration of this lesion help in the diagnosis?

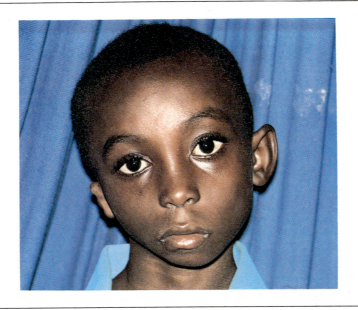

Q 6.14 (a) What condition is illustrated here?

      (b) What is the cause?

      (c) Which facial structures are primarily affected?

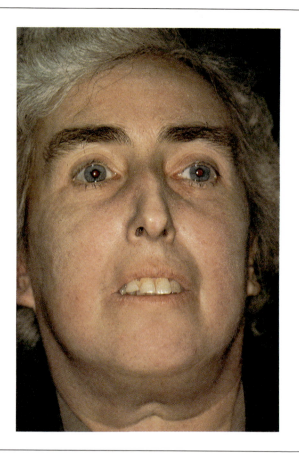

Q 6.15 This 55 year old lady had some difficulties during dental treatment because she found it difficult to open her mouth widely.

(a) What is the probable diagnosis?

(b) What specific changes might dental radiography demonstrate?

(c) What salivary pathology may be present?

A 6.1 (a) Herpes zoster (shingles).
Crusted lesions are confined to the distribution of the maxillary division of the trigeminal nerve — characteristic of shingles.

(b) Herpes varicella-zoster virus: this virus causes chicken-pox and then remains latent in the dorsal root ganglia but is reactivated if there is immune depression, for example in old age, in the immunosuppressed patient, or if there is an underlying neoplasm.

(c) (i) Severe oral ulceration (ipsilateral palate and upper vestibule).
(ii) Severe pain.
(iii) Post-herpetic neuralgia: this may be so severe and intractable as to cause depression.

NB Chickenpox on forehead. Some patients with zoster also have chickenpox lesions.

A 6.2 Nasopalatine cyst.

This cyst is just behind the incisive papilla and originates from epithelium of the nasopalatine canal. The nasopalatine cyst is considered by many to be the most common of the developmental oral cysts. There is no sex predilection and the cyst often remains undetected although it may be revealed radiographically. Usually asymptomatic but if infection occurs an abscess results.

A 6.3 (a) Black hairy tongue. The middle of the dorsum of the tongue shows a black hairy appearance caused by elongated filiform papillae.

(b) (i) Antibiotics (penicillin or tetracycline).
(ii) Mouthwashes (sodium perborate or chlorhexidine).
(iii) Iron preparations.
(iv) Smoking.
(v) Some foodstuffs.

(c) (i) Discontinuing the causal factors if known.
(ii) Brushing the tongue.
(iii) Sucking a peach stone!

A 6.4 (a) (i) Hereditary angioneurotic oedema (HANE)
(ii) Allergy to some dental material or drug (angioedema).

(b) (i) HANE — estimation of serum C1 esterase inhibitor (which is reduced in this condition) and serum complement levels (C3 and C4).
(ii) Referral for allergy testing.

(c) Airways obstruction as a consequence of lingual and laryngeal oedema. In some families with HANE up to one third succumb.

HANE is a rare autosomal dominant condition in which trauma (often minor) precipitates uncontrolled complement activation and oedema particularly of the head and neck. Patients have a deficiency of, or a defect of, an inhibitor of the complement system (C1 esterase inhibitor).

Drug allergies in dentistry are usually to penicillin, or to one of the intravenous anaesthetic agents. Allergies to local analgesics (lignocaine and prilocaine) are very, very rare, although patients may react to another component of the solution such as the paramino benzoic acid preservative.

Allergy to dental materials is rare but there are well-documented instances of reactions to eugenol or other essential oils, to various impression materials and to various dental filling materials such as the epoxy resins. However, true allergy to denture materials is almost unheard of: most reactions are to free monomer or are quite unrelated to the denture.

In established HANE dental treatment should only be carried out in hospital after pre-treatment with danazol or stanazol, and possibly antifibrinolytic agents.

A 6.5 (a) There is smoker's keratosis (stomatitis nicotina) in the palate — but also a carcinoma in the retromolar region!

(b) (i) Biopsy to establish diagnosis. In this type of case, both the neoplasm and the keratotic soft palate should be biopsied.

(ii) Management of the neoplasm depends on extent of local spread and lymph node metastasis. Radiotherapy is usually the treatment of choice in established lesions in this site and the irradiated field may be planned to include the remainder of the soft palate to eliminate the keratosis. Surgery may be indicated if there is evidence of bony involvement, and combination therapy of surgery followed by radiotherapy may also be instituted. The patient should be discouraged from further smoking.

Smoker's keratosis is typified by a diffuse white lesion of the palate in which the orifices of the minor salivary glands appear as pink spots as shown here. Usually caused by pipe smoking, smoker's keratosis is commonly benign. However, as shown here, it is vital to exclude any other more serious lesions. Smoker's keratosis may resolve if smoking is stopped.

For further discussion on oral carcinoma see A5.4 and A2.4.

A 6.6 (a) (i) The patient should be asked to swallow. Thyroglossal lesions will be seen to move up with the thyroid cartilage.

(ii) Aspiration with a wide bore needle. If the aspirate obtained is of a straw-coloured fluid, then a thyroglossal cyst may be suspected. This swelling may possibly represent a mucous extravasation cyst such as a ranula and gelatinous fluid will be aspirated. Such a midline swelling is unlikely to arise from a lymph node, but any of the lymphomas may be the cause. When this particular lesion was aspirated, it became obvious that this represented a solid lesion of some sort. Histological examination of material contained within the needle confirmed that it was keratin.

(iii) Incisional biopsy. Aspiration will usually confirm the diagnosis in this sort of case, but should the lesion be solid in nature then a neoplasm should be suspected and a biopsy performed.

These simple investigations will usually clarify the diagnosis. If one of the lymphomas is suspected, then appropriate further investigations should be performed. Computerized axial tomography or ultrasonic examination will confirm the extent of this lesion.

(b) 1. Ranula.
2. Thyroglossal cyst.
3. Implantation dermoid cyst.
4. Lymphoma or other neoplasm.

A careful history revealed that the patient had sustained a penetrating injury to the submandibular skin at the age of 4 years from a broken milk bottle. This implantation dermoid cyst had obviously been slowly growing for more than 50 years. This slow growth explained her lack of symptoms. The accompanying picture shows the enucleated specimen which was retrieved via an intraoral approach and midline division of the tongue (Fig. A6.6).

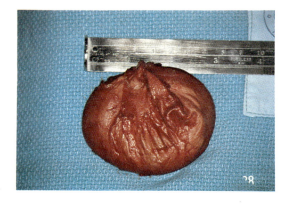

Fig. A6.6

A 6.7 (a) Ranula. This mucous extravasation cyst takes its name from the Latin for 'little frog' in that the overlying mucosa is very thin and shows clearly the mucosal vasculature. The cause of these lesions is trauma to the ducts of the sublingual salivary gland such that a breach is produced which allows saliva to escape into the tissues.

(b) Anteriorly, the mylohoid muscle limits the inferior extension of these lesions, and the tongue will be displaced upwards by the increasingly large volume of mucus. Posteriorly, ranulas arising from the posterior aspect of the sublingual gland have no limiting anatomical structure inferiorly and may extend several inches downwards into the neck. This condition is then described as a 'plunging ranula'.

(c) These extravasation cysts have no epithelial lining and will regress if the cause is removed. This involves excision of the offending sublingual salivary gland. It is not necessary to remove every last millilitre of viscid saliva from the plunging variety as this will be dealt with by macrophages.

NB $\overline{\text{E}}|$ is retained.

A 6.8 (a) (i) There is a well defined area of radiolucency affecting the right ascending ramus of mandible, superimposed on $7|$ indicating that the lesion here occupies the bone buccal to this tooth (lingual bone is usually thin). This lesion is limited posteriorly and inferiorly by the inferior dental bundle which nevertheless has been displaced backwards and downwards (as compared with the other side).
   (ii) Unerupted $|3$.
   (iii) Submerged $|\text{E}$ or supplemental premolar $|45$ region.
   (iv) Retained $|\text{C}$.
   (v) Small area of radiopacity associated with mesial root of $|6$.

(b) No. The vast majority of impacted upper canines can be localized by simple inspection and palpation. Teeth not palpable by this means are usually in the line of the arch when no amount of radiographs will move them labially or palatally!

   Further periapical radiographs may be useful however in determining root morphology, condition of retained deciduous canines and the presence of resorption affecting the permanent incisors. Clearly, in this case, periapical views will be necessary to examine further the other buried tooth in this quadrant.

(c) $\overline{8|}$ is displaced to the level of the sigmoid notch by the cystic lesion in the ramus. Both upper third molars appear to be in a normal position as does the $\overline{|8}$. Assessment of third molars radiographically depends on an appreciation of the normal development of third molars. There is a temptation to say that $\overline{|8}$ is impacted, but third molars commonly occupy such a position developmentally. Indeed, the spacing between $\overline{|34}$ indicates an absence of crowding in this quadrant.

A 6.9 (a) The two major causes of anterior open-bite are habits such as thumb-sucking and vertical skeletal anomalies. The face height can be measured easily by comparing the proportions of the lower and middle thirds of the face, which should be roughly equal.

(b) This appearance is most unlikely to be due to a pathological process. In the World Health Organisation classification of disease, malocclusions like this one are termed anomalies rather than pathological conditions.

(c) Anterior open-bite.

NB $\underline{2|}$ is absent and $\underline{1|1}$ are crowned teeth.

A 6.10 (a) Hand, foot and mouth disease.

(b) Coxsackie viruses A_{16} usually.

(c) Children usually: it is fairly contagious.

Oral ulcers have many causes (see Answers to Questions 1.6, 1.8, 1.10, 2.6, 2.13, 3.4, 4.9, 4.11, 5.4, 5.9, 5.15, and 6.1). Of the infective causes, viral infections are the most frequent infections that produce mouth ulcers. Herpes simplex stomatitis, chicken-pox, herpangina, zoster, and infectious mononucleosis are the viral infections most likely to produce ulcers. The ulcers shown here are not pathognomonic: similar ulcers may appear in any of these viral disorders. However, the cutaneous vesicles point to the diagnosis of hand, foot and mouth disease.

A 6.11 (a) Gorlin's syndrome. (Gorlin–Goltz or Basal Cell Naevoid syndrome).

(b) Skull radiograph (calcified falx cerebri); chest radiograph (bifid ribs and other abnormalities).

Gorlin's syndrome is the association of multiple odontogenic keratocysts, multiple cutaneous basal cell carcinomas (shown here) and multiple skeletal abnormalities.

An autosomal dominant condition, Gorlin's syndrome manifests with frontal and temporoparietal bossing, mild ocular hypertelorism and mild mandibular prognathism.

Cutaneous lesions are basal cell carcinomas and, on the palms and soles, a peculiar dyskeratosis.

Jaw cysts usually appear in childhood or adolescence and have a particular tendency to recur after surgery.

Vertebral anomalies include bifid or splayed ribs, kyphoscoliosis, vertebral anomalies, short fourth metacarpal bones, and various minor abnormalities.

A 6.12 (a) Denture granuloma (epulis fissuratum). The horizontal fissure in this lesion indicates the position of the labial flange of the upper full denture. These lesions may present as vascular granulomatous lesions or established fibrous lesions.

(b) The upper denture should be widely relieved in the first instance. Alternatively, the denture should not be worn at all. Withdrawal of the irritant responsible for this condition will often lead to a striking reduction in the size of the swelling. Very often, early lesions will resolve completely by this simple measure. Established fibrotic lesions and large lesions such as this one will require surgical excision of remaining tissue after a period of approximately three months. It is important that any surgical reduction of this tissue is not accompanied by avoidable reduction in labial sulcus depth leading to difficulty with the wearing of upper dentures in the future.

(c) These lesions have no propensity to undergo malignant change but, very rarely, a similar appearance may arise if a neoplasm enlarges to encroach upon a denture flange.

NB Sinus in 54| region proved to be caused by a retained root.

A 6.13 (a) There is evidence of a multilocular lesion affecting the anterior part of the mandible. This may be an ameloblastoma (adamantinoma), an odontogenic myxoma, or a multilocular keratocyst. None of these lesions usually gives rise to infiltration of adjacent sensory nerves leading to paraesthesia or anaesthesia. The two locally invasive tumours (ameloblastoma and odontogenic myxoma) may however give rise to resorption of adjacent teeth.

(b) A measure of total protein content of aspirate from ameloblas-
tomas typically shows a level greater than 5 g/100 ml of fluid.
This concentration is similar to that obtained from other
odontogenic cysts apart from the keratocyst which typically
shows a level lower than 4 g/100 ml. These conditions can thus
be differentiated by this means. No aspirate is normally
obtained from a myxoma.

A 6.14 (a) Hemifacial microsomia (first and second branchial arch syndrome, Oculoauriculovertebral dysplasia) affecting the right
side.

(b) Haematoma arising from the stapedial artery *in utero*. This
artery, vestigial in nature after birth, is the artery of the second
branchial arch. Occlusion of this vessel and organization of an
adjacent haematoma before development of the branchial arch
has been completed will give rise to lack of growth and
differentiation of adjacent structures. This growth defect can be
associated with anomalies affecting heart, kidney, and skeleton
and this, allied to an hereditary component, is evidence of the
operation of other aetiological factors apart from haematoma
formation.

(c) This abnormality in growth affects structures arising
from Meckel's cartilage, including the ossicles, glenoid fossa,
mandibular condyle, ascending ramus, body of mandible, and
associated structures such as masseter, medial pterygoid, and
pinna. These manifestations often give rise to striking
asymmetry, particularly if maxillary, temporal and zygomatic
bones are affected. Approximately 10 per cent of patients with
this deformity demonstrate bilateral involvement, and frontal
bone bossing may also be a feature. The severity of deformity
appears to depend on the exact time of stapedial artery
occlusion and extent of haematoma, and there may, therefore,
be very variable effects on both affected bone and soft tissue.
Thorough examination to evaluate associated skeletal, cardiac,
and renal anomalies should be performed.

A 6.15 (a) Systemic sclerosis.

(b) In a minority of patients (8–10 per cent) there is widening of
the periodontal space.

(c) Sjögren's syndrome (see A1.15).

This disease, of uncertain aetiology, affects predominantly the connective tissue and may cause trismus since the skin (including facial skin) becomes tight, giving the face an unwrinkled 'Mona Lisa' appearance.

The tongue also may be firm and develop a 'chicken tongue' appearance. Oral telangiectasia may develop — as shown (Fig. A6.15(i)). Raynaud's phenomenon may complicate systemic sclerosis and produce digital ischaemia and subsequent necrosis, as shown here (Fig. A6.15(ii)).

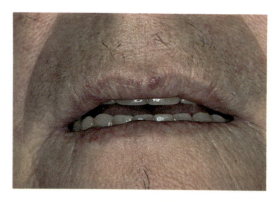

Fig. A6.15(i)

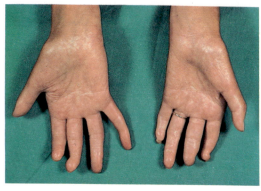

Fig. A6.15(ii)

References

Cawson, R. A. (1984). *Essentials of Dental Surgery and Pathology* Churchill Livingstone, Edinburgh.

Cawson, R. A. and Scully, C. (1985). *MCQ's in Dentistry* Churchill Livingstone, Edinburgh.

Cawson, R. A., Scully, C. and Yap, P. L. (1986). *Aids to Clinical Immunology*. Churchill Livingstone, Edinburgh.

Dolby, A. E., Walker, D. M. and Matthews, N. (1981). *Introduction to Oral Immunology*. Arnold, London.

Gorlin, R. J. and Goldman, H. M. (1970). *Oral Pathology (Thoma's Oral Pathology)*. Mosby, Louis, Missouri.

Jones, J. H. and Mason, D. K. (1980). *Oral Manifestations of Systemic Disease*. Saunders, London.

Scully, C. (1985). *Hospital Dental Surgeon's Guide*. British Dental Association, London.

Scully, C. and Cawson, R. A. (1982). *Medical Problems in Dentistry*. Wright, PSG, London.

Scully, C. and Cawson, R. A. (1986). *Oral Medicine*. Medicine International, Oxford.

Subject Index